I0413556

THIS BOOK IS MADE POSSIBLE BY THE UNSELFISH CONTRIBUTIONS OF MANY ORDINARY AND PROFESSIONAL PEOPLE WHO COMBINED TO ENSURE THAT THE WORLD BECOMES A BETTER PLACE THROUGH THE SHARING OF KNOWLEDGE...

MAY THIS BOOK ALWAYS CONTINUE TO BUILD ON THIS INTENTION...

Go and buy a copy of African dream by Vicky Sampson and let her voice inspire you... It inspired NELSON MANDELA while he was President of South Africa... It played as I needed inspiration to finish this book as I reached the deadline on Sunday 9th March 2014and I was still writing hard... But I will finish this on time. Today is that time...

FETAL ALCOHOL SYNDROME   SPECIAL LAUNCH EDITION

ISBN-13: 978 – 149615 7867   ISBN-10: 149 615 7869

MY CROSS TO BEAR

THE TRUE HEART–RENDING STORIES OF INNOCENT VICTIMS AND
THE HELPLESS PERPETRATORS IN THIS EXPOSE`

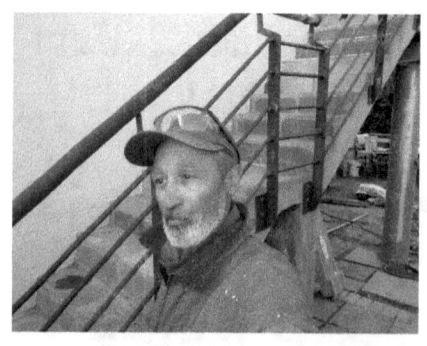
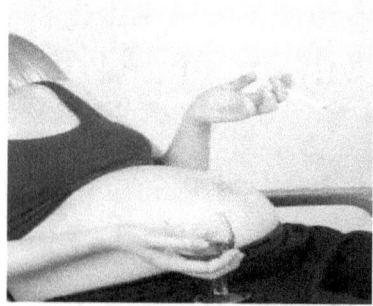

BY HENRY AFRICA   2

5 FACTORS THAT LEAD TO FAS

FACTOR 1: LACK OF NATIONAL AWARENESS CAMPAIGN
No knowledge about potential dangers facing pregnant women

FACTOR 2: LACK OF PRE-NATAL EDUCATION
Should one obtain a license to have children first?

FACTOR 3: DRINKING & DRUGS DURING PREGNANCY
Ingesting harmful toxins of various kinds-alcohol is one

FACTOR 4: A CHID GRANT SYSTEM WITHOUT EDUCATION
An incentive to earn money results in some unloved children

FACTOR 5: LACK OF A PREGNANCY REGISTER
A nation should care about every citizen who is about to be born

What right have I got as male and as author to label this a **CRIME**? Am I inviting judgment by society on **HELPLESS and** addicted individuals who want nothing more than an extension of themselves, that they can love and help to have a better life, than they are living or would like to live? How much do I really care if I am creating an environment wherein people start to judge each other and cast stones when they need to take the plank out of their own eyes first? But maybe you need to turn this conversation around for a while.

"HOW CAN WE CONTINUE TO STAND BY WHILE INNOCENT CHILDREN ARE BROUGHT INTO THIS WORLD DEFORMED WITH PRIOR KNOWLDEGE ABOUT THE DANGERS INVOLVED IN THEIR CREATION?"

Then we have to help the perpetrators to cope with the consequences as a society when we watched them create the mess they were about to suffer through… And that suffering would involve us for the rest of the victim's lives? If I was the VICTIM then I would ask…

"WHY DID YOU DO NOTHING TO PREVENT THIS FROM HAPPENING?"
DID YOU CARE SO LITTLE FOR MY FUTURE?

WOULD IT BE OK TO REPLY…"I AM SORRY BUT I DIDN'T KNOW WHAT WAS HAPPENING TO YOU?"

BY HENRY AFRICA   **3**

PROLOGUE

THE HISTORY OF FAS [FETAL ALCOHOL SYNDROME]

A group of doctors first noticed that there were a specific set of circumstances around a group who had been treated for s specific condition. They started using the term Fetal Alcohol Syndrome Disorder around that time.

It is generally accepted that Fetal Alcohol Syndrome is 100% preventable. Translated that means that there is no reason for any child to be born with an alcohol related disease or for an adult to have to be living with the side effects of this type of condition. It has been dismissed as a genetic condition and so is not inherited by any succeeding generation even from the parent who may have been born with the condition. That means that a person diagnosed with FASD can have a completely healthy child if only they did not partake of alcohol during their pregnancy or from the time they are diagnosed to be pregnant.

This would make this disorder one that is completely in the hands of the women who have an alcohol and drug addiction and who subsequently fall pregnant. It therefore means that the male chromosome has nothing to do with the resultant disorder in any way. It is directly attributed to the ingestation of alcohol during the pregnancy of the woman and is a completely avoidable event that will carry a life sentence for both the soon-to-be-born victim and the female perpetrator. They will spend a lifetime together living through the hell of the perpetrators own choosing. Alcohol will have the final say in this episode. Do drugs play a role? Abstain from one drug then have to abstain from all, besides adopting a healthy diet. Then you give your unborn child every chance to be born healthy…

GOAL OF THIS BOOK
BREAKING THE CYCLE

Breaking the cycle refers to the habit of drinking excessively. Can you harness a snake and not let it bite you when it has the opportunity? Can you harness the rain and use the water when you need it? Can you store the wind and make it available when you need the energy most? The answer is yes... To each one of those questions the answer is yes... Now I hear some people say...
"What he been smoking lately?" and others say
"Maybe he has been harvesting some home-grown weed of his own"

The general majority will know that all things are possible today, in 2014 as I write this book. But it was not that way back 30 or 40 years ago was it?

How can a guy spend 20 days in a cage and not get bitten by a snake when the cage is filled with them? Poisonous snakes amongst the lot? How long ago was it that we did not have the dam technology that we have today?

We are capable of building wind farms and storing the electricity before we need to use it. We feed it into a grid that adds to the electricity we have stored. Yes is the answer to the questions. But, would the answer be yes if we were standing in the year 1652? Guess then the answer would have to be NO right...

So can we conquer Fetal Alcohol Syndrome? Guess you agree now with me if I said the answer is yes right? And you would be right...

YES WE CAN BREAK THE CYCLE... YES IT IS GOING TO HAPPEN...In our lifetime IT CAN BECOME A REALITY...YES?

BY HENRY AFRICA

DEDICATED TO
A FEW PEOPLE WHO TRULY CARE

You can find some people who care on this websites. They will try to help you in any way they can. But it is really up to you to make sure that you prevent this EVENT from happening to you...www.FASiceberg.org

I was first alerted to the problems around FASD during a ROUTINE VISIT TO THE DEPARTMENT WHERE SUBMISSIONS TO CITY LIBRARIES TAKES PLACE. That was about 5 years ago, in 2009. I had just published a book on Relationships & Conflict Management... Staying Happily Married Is Hard But Not Impossible. It can be obtained on Amazon.com too...
"We have lots of books on this relationship topic," The lady had said. I doubt we can take one more. But I will submit it anyway," she added.
"This is the lead book and a new way of teaching subject matter. Pictures and content education..." I had said to her... She didn't get it at that time... Meg & Spiky, a new education subject's time had yet to come... My struggle was not over yet...But I would not quit... Winners never quit do they!!...

Well they didn't accept it for circulation then. Perhaps they should have. It will help you communicate more effectively with your FAS child too. I never really heard what she said after that, or really was too engrossed in marketing the book I had written. To start a new book after spending 20 000zar on the one I had just completed was not on my agenda. 5 years later I have seen the potential need... A book about FASD is needed. Then I remembered what that lady had said... **"If you write a book on FETAL ALCOHOL SYNDROME then I would take it**. I did not have a clue what FAS was at the time...A new way of looking at this situation is needed... A book that WILL help millions to understand the depths of despair involved in this hidden tragedy within our societies...

A chat with my friend Fergus O'Connor, has led me to commit to write a book that perhaps will help highlight the challenges many parents face. This is a partnership to help many people. Because Fergus really does care... About parents who struggle with children who are slow learners... About friends who are in difficult situations... About family who hot tough patches... My childhood friend has taught me to care more too. Care enough to sacrifice my time for others a little more. Some of them may have suffered with FAS symptoms. They never even knew this because they were fighting a system that kept them in the dark. But we are the masters of the system. We need to take action to change systems... INFORMATION IS POWER...

Some parents face their struggles alone... I hope my contribution will make a difference... It is a heart rending decision to raise this FAS child as your own when you adopt. You need to be brave and you need to know you cannot do this alone... You need the help of God or the journey will be too much for you to bear... My heart goes out to each and every parent of every child who suffers with this disorder. It does not matter how it happened... If it happened in ignorance then it happened... Moving on as they say... Action is need to fix and to repair a system that is inadequate to cope with a situation that is escalating and may be out of control if we do not put some newly developed controls in place...

But if you are ignorant of this subject, then you are not alone. There are millions of people who have walked this road. There are millions who WILL walk this road in the future. Your concern about the future of your child and also the future of that child's own children is one you have reason to be concerned about. Your God has heard your prayers. He waits to help you through the pain you are about to face as the parent of an FAS child. It's His child too... "OUR FATHER WHICH ART IN HEAVEN... PLEASE HELP US..." And God has heard their prayers...

Society is largely drug dependent. Cigarettes, alcohol, cocaine, heroin, crystal meths, LSD, rocks, prescription pain killers. Sadly it is getting worse as we speak, not better. Yes, we want it to get better but we face a brushfire of sorts in curbing crime, drug abuse, substance abuses and incurable diseases... Cancer, Alzheimers, Parkinsons, Leukemia etc. etc. Oh yeah then there is that thing called FASD. It has been placed at the end of the disorder food-chain. It is a huge problem and we have only begun to see the TIP OF THE ICEBERG. This is the best I can do to help right now...

GOD WILL INSPIRE ME AS I WRITE THIS BOOK. The stories shared may bring tears to the eyes of those who have lived with the problems around this subject ALL their lives. It is my goal to help READERS feel the pain felt by millions. They have been shouldering that pain alone... It is time we truly understood to what depth this problem impacts our society... It is time we really as a world take a deeper interest in something we have been watching but really doing very little about... Is that a fair accusation to make? Could we have really been ignoring the suffering of millions? Yes! We do it in many ways as a society... We do it with poverty stricken children all over the world... Kids run around with bloated bellies and we still simply get up and go to work... We say..."There is nothing I can do about it" And then we say... "One man or woman can make a difference"... Isn't that true?

BOOK OUTLINE

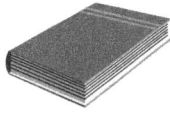

CONTENTS

CHAPTER **1** ONE

WHO SAID ITS FETAL ALCOHOL SYNDROME

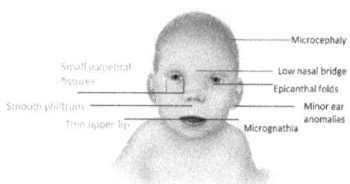

How do you know that I have Fetal Alcohol Syndrome? Maybe I am just born this way? Maybe I was always going to look like this? Can you simply label me by association? Can you do that?

She looks pretty ordinary to me. Attractive too. Depends on what her character is like. That other model from Cosmopolitan was rude compared to Richelle. And Richelle is great company too. Has a hot body. You must just see her in a bikini…She is to die for…

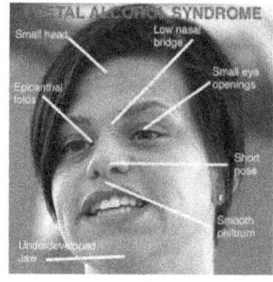

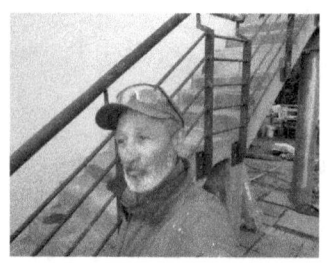

OBSERVATION

Preconceived ideas are unhealthy... Assuming that FAS sufferers are inferior may leave you with egg on your face. Lose the superior complex and treat ALL people equally.

IT'S THE BEST WAY TO LIVE...

SUMMARY

Why my child God? Why did it have to happen to my child? I did nothing Lord. I have always been a good person. Good things happened to bad people too. Bad things happen to good people too. Would you really·like to know why you were chosen to go through this ordeal?

BECAUSE YOU ARE STRONG ENOUGH…AND SPECIAL ENOUGH TO HANDLE IT…

BY HENRY AFRICA

"BEAUTY LIES BURIED BENEATH THE SHELL FOR THE BEHOLDER. AND GOD SEES THE HEART"

By Henry Africa

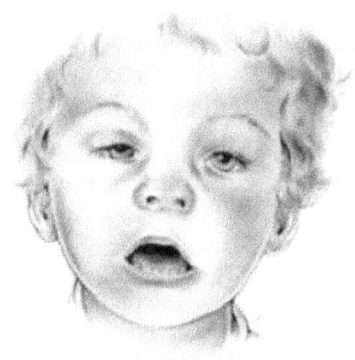

WHY MAKE ME DIFFERENT GOD. DO YOU HATE ME SO MUCH?

NO, IT'S BECAUSE I LOVE YOU SO MUCH THAT I HAVE MADE YOU SPECIAL. DO YOU LOVE YOURSELF ENOUGH TO FIND OUT HOW STRONG YOU REALLY ARE? STRONG ENOUGH TO OVERCOME EVEN THIS CHALLENGE?

CAN YOU TRUST ME ENOUGH TO BEAR YOUR CROSS AND THEN SPEND AN ETERNITY WITH ME? WELL? YES? WILL YOU?

CHAPTER 1 ONE

WHO SAID ITS FETAL ALCOHOL SYNDROME

Who defined the term **ALCOHOL FETAL SYNDROME**? Who gave the name to a group and called them Nigger, Coolie, Maori, Aborigine, Coloreds? Was it God inspired?

Is this group name in the interest of the child or adult? Does the group's self esteem improve by being associated with this group name? Does it segregate in a positive way? Or does it not just alienate one group from others and invite them to be treated differently from the rest

FETAL ACOHOL SYNDROME SUFFERER. Is that all I will be remembered for one day? Now that is a question that only you can answer for yourself. They can place a tag on you and call you a DUCK. But if you are a SWAN then a SWAN you will remain. If you are a bird then fly you will. And if you were meant to be something special then nothing can stop that or can it?

SUMMARY

I am not about to lay into the medical fraternity. They love to label things and then carry on to label people too. Species have been documented for millions of years. Criminals will be tagged then feathered, tarred and set alight. If you lived in the year 1500 it was possible. Who governs the tagging system? No the doctors I can say…

Who says the tag Doctor is a superior one? Who says the tag golfer is one to strive for? What about tennis player? Lawyer? They are all tags attached to people. So I have FAS. It WILL NOT stop me from becoming one of the best humans possible. I can achieve any goal I set for myself. If the road to the top is a little more difficult because of that tag then bring it on. I will fight any obstacle in my path and rise to the top in whatever field I am going to put my hand to. I am a winner and not even FAS will stand in the way of my success. I just need patient sensitive people around me who will take the time to care… IT IS SAID**…"PEOPLE DON'T CARE HOW MUCH YOU KNOW UNTIL THEY KNOW HOW MUCH YOU CARE**… And I want to encourage you to care…Care about those with tags who have a tough time bearing the cross society attaches to them…

Now that will make you a special human being in the eyes of the one who really matters...God is only one who needs to be impressed by you…What people say and do will not matter in the greater scheme of things… Time will pass and then so will people too… Only what we say will be remembered by God and shown to us some far-off day in the future. Did we do what was right? That is the question we have to answer every day and if we can say yes then we WILL be ok…

CHAPTER *2* TWO
SOCIETY SHOUTS SO SILENTLY

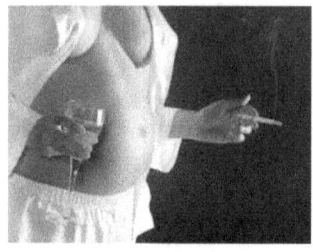

I know I will be strung up if I am caught drinking like this while I am obviously pregnant. But I have tried so many times to quit this habit and find it almost impossible. I just don't have the willpower to carry it through. Maybe I need to get some help from a group of some kind...

I will need to read up about this potential problem. If I do want to have a child then I will need to make certain sacrifices to ensure that my child is born healthy. Boozing is one of them.

I must be prepared to make the sacrifices. It's my responsibility...Oh and my party habit may need to go for a while too...

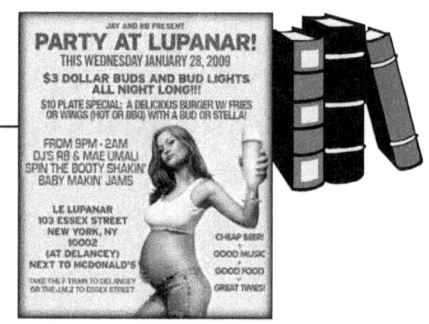

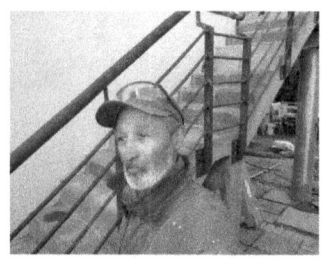

Society finds it easy to condemn. But society first needs to understand before it decides to condemn. There are reasons we have got into the position we are in with regard to lots of things. Rather than judge each other, we need to HELP each other to try and be better human beings before we choose the easy way out and judge...

SUMMARY:

It is sometimes difficult to have to stand up for what is right. Especially if you have to stand up in a society where it seems like you are the only one who is passionate enough to show the resolve to stand up.

But if your life is judged by what you have done to make the world a better place then you HAVE TO just do what is right...In Gods eyes. And let God help you as you go along...

"ALL OUR DREAMS CAN COME TRUE IF WE JUST PERSUE THEM"

"PERSISTANCE PAYS OFF"

Walt Elias Disney
[Born 1905]

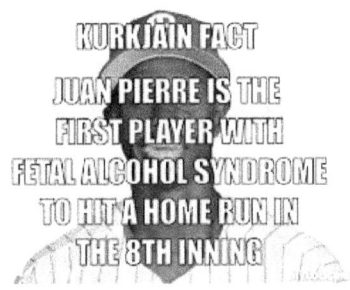

BECOME A SPORTS STAR

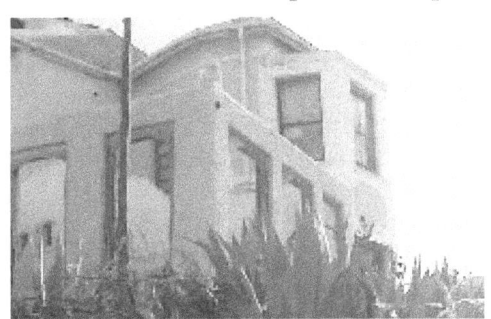

BUY A HOUSE AND RENOVATE IT

DO NOT LET THE FEAR OF THE UNKNOWN STOP YOU FROM GOING AFTER WHAT MAY APPEAR TO BE AN IMPOSSIBLE DREAM.

Here I can draw a parallel with many top sportspeople who have had to overcome serious hurdles before they have reached the pinnacle of their sport of choice. Look at the picture above...

Is it going to be any different for you if you have one of a range of diseases? NO! It is going to be tough if you have ADHD or Alzheimers, Parkinsons... YES even FASD is one of them too.

YOU WILL HAVE TO BE STRONG AND COURAGEOUS OR YOU WILL NOT MANAGE TO REALIZE YOUR LIFE GOALS.

AND YOU NEED TO HAVE A LIFE GOAL. NO MATTER IF YOU ARE HEALTHY OR SUFFERING FROM ANY ONE OF A DOZEN DIFFERENT CHALLENGING DISORDERS...

CHAPTER2TWO

SOCIETY SHOUTS SO SILENTLY

Megan is pregnant and she does not want to listen to us about the danger that her continued drinking poses to her unborn child. Will she only remember what we tried to tell her once she has to live with a child that has been diagnosed with Fetal Alcohol Syndrome? Why is it that women do not yet see that their newborn babies can be affected by the booze and the drugs that they ingest during the 9 months of pregnancy? If they really are serious about having a child that is born healthy, then they should abstain from drinking during their 9 months of pregnancy. Is there anything we can do to help the baby? Ultimately the child will suffer if it is born deformed due to its mother's stubbornness with regards to quitting this practice for even the short period of 9 months.

We have all spoken to her as friends. What else can we do to make her listen to us? Must we lodge a lawsuit against her and get the courts to stop her from abusing her fetus? It is as close to murder as you can get. Sadly the fetus does not yet have the rights that it should in our world. If it did then we may be able to get legal help to stop what she is doing. Her drinking and abuse of substance is going to help produce a deformed child. She goes out every weekend and does not come home until the next day…What about Mandy. She and her husband do drugs and booze all weekend but come Monday, they become model citizens, and stay that way till Friday… Social alcoholic is a term we would use to describe them… We can try and help but we cannot force them... Can we…? Do we want to?

SUMMARY:

What can I say to make you feel any better? We have not taken our responsibilities as a society to the point where we can protect a fetus from abuse... Not yet anyway. We are still trying to get to the point where we can protect our innocent children from abuse. Some parents have been found guilty of burning their babies… Have been found guilty of raping their male and female children… How can we as a society protect a fetus if we cannot yet protect a child that has already been born?

We can only hope that by improving our education system we can solve problems like this. Preventative education that achieves the goal of educating against dangers like alcohol and drugs. We as a society face dangers from the very drugs that have been designed to help us. ABUSE of drugs and alcohol, leads to children who are not born the way they should have been. Responsible use of drugs is the solution to this problem...

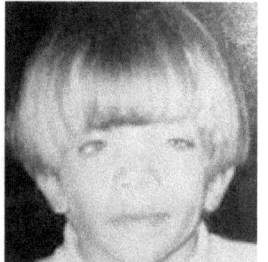

100% PREVENTABLE

CHAPTER 3 THREE

COULDN'T YOU ABSTAIN FOR JUST 9 MONTHS

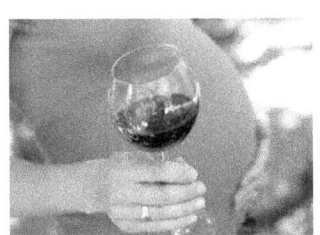

What will it mean for me to do without the usual glass of wine? Nothing wrong with turning the usual glass of wine into a usual glass of fruit juice or mineral water.

It's entirely a habit that has been acquired from our parents. I know that I can do without it if I really try…

"The child I am going to be depends to a large degree on what you do during the 9 months you are pregnant, Mom Yes, you can carry on with your party lifestyle but you are risking my chances of being born a healthy baby…"

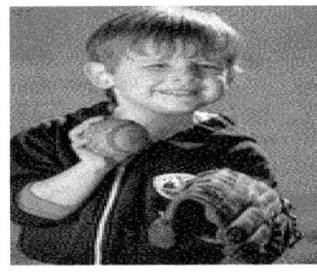

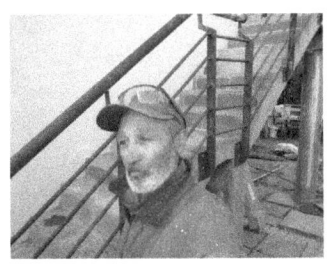

The wine company will not go bankrupt if you don't buy the usual bottle of wine. The grape farmer will survive too. You can return to your usual glass of, wine, after a meal, when you have given birth to a sparkling healthy child… Is it that too much to sacrifice?

SUMMARY:

You may go through 9months of pregnancy and give birth to a healthy baby, even if you are drinking your usual glass of wine every night or a few times a week. You may have done that in the past, but was the wine you drink now, as high in alcohol content as before? Nowadays the wine alcohol level is higher in many wines…Do you check that?

"IT WILL NOT HARM YOU TO GIVE THE WINE COMPANY A MISS FOR THE 9 MONTHS OF YOUR PREGNANCY…"

"I HAVE ONE LIFE TO LIVE; I AM NOT GOING TO NEGATIVELY AFFECT MY UNBORN CHILD'S LIFE DUE TO ALCOHOL OR DRUGS"

ANONOMOUS

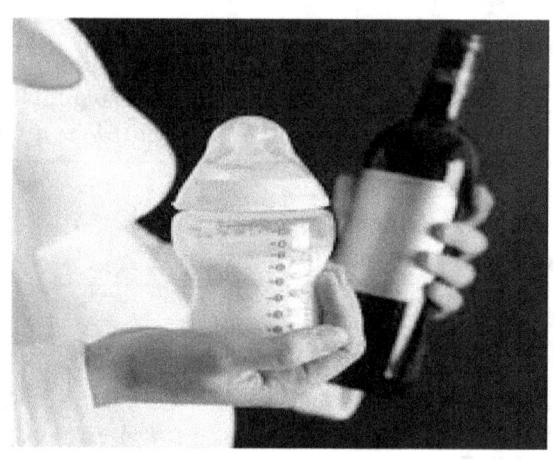

CONVICT YOURSELF OF THE NEED TO ABSTAIN BY READING UP ON THE SUBJECT OF FETAL ALCOHOL SYNDROME... DON'T SIMPLY TAKE MY WORD FOR IT...

It is a responsibility you have towards your unborn child. You have to read up on lots of things so that you ensure that your child is given every opportunity to be born healthy...

EVERYTHING you eat and drink is shared by your unborn child. That includes ALL food and beverages you consume. Make sure you are giving your unborn child the best possible products... Quality products...

BY HENRY AFRICA   **18**

CHAPTER 3 THREE

COULDN'T YOU ABSTAIN FOR 9 MONTHS

I know that my friends judge me because they are aware that I am still drinking even though I am already 6 months pregnant. They have been preaching to me at every opportunity since I shared the wonderful news of my pregnancy.

I know it is dangerous for my unborn child but I just cannot stop drinking. I have been a social alcoholic for my whole life. They called me the life and soul of the party but now they do not even invite me to any of the parties they host. I know they are trying to help me, to stop being tempted by alcohol, by not inviting me but it means I have found other friends who are simply too glad to have me around over weekends and they buy all the drink I need.

And the guys buy me booze at every opportunity. Guess they appreciate that I will do anything for a drink. I may as well be honest and tell you that I will sell my soul for a drink. Sleeping with a guy is a small price to pay to get what I cannot do without… It is impossible for me to go without alcohol for even a day…

SUMMARY:

SHAME!!! We are so sooo sorry for you. And yes, I want that to sound the way it should. Sorry, I cannot go without abusing my unborn baby even for one day. I cannot go without beating my unborn child just a few times. I used to beat the child only once or twice a day. Now that I know it is wrong I beat the child every few days.

Does that sound crazy to you too? How can you beat the child even once? There is a difference between beating the child and disciplining the child. Killing the child just a little bit every day? Is that acceptable to you? Deforming my unborn child just a little bit every day for 9 months? Is that acceptable to us as a society? That is what you doing when you drink alcohol during your pregnancy.

It is no longer a research project. The conclusions have been medically established. Perhaps you may have been ignorant about this for your whole life. I was not aware of the seriousness of this subject until I wrote this book. I am male and so I do not have the same responsibility when it comes to having children. But that is the way it has been put out by God. Women are the ones who have to carry the children. Men can only show support during the 9 month process. And if they do not? Can you blame them for what you do?

CHAPTER 4 FOUR
DID I MATTER SO LITTLE TO YOU THAT YOU DRANK

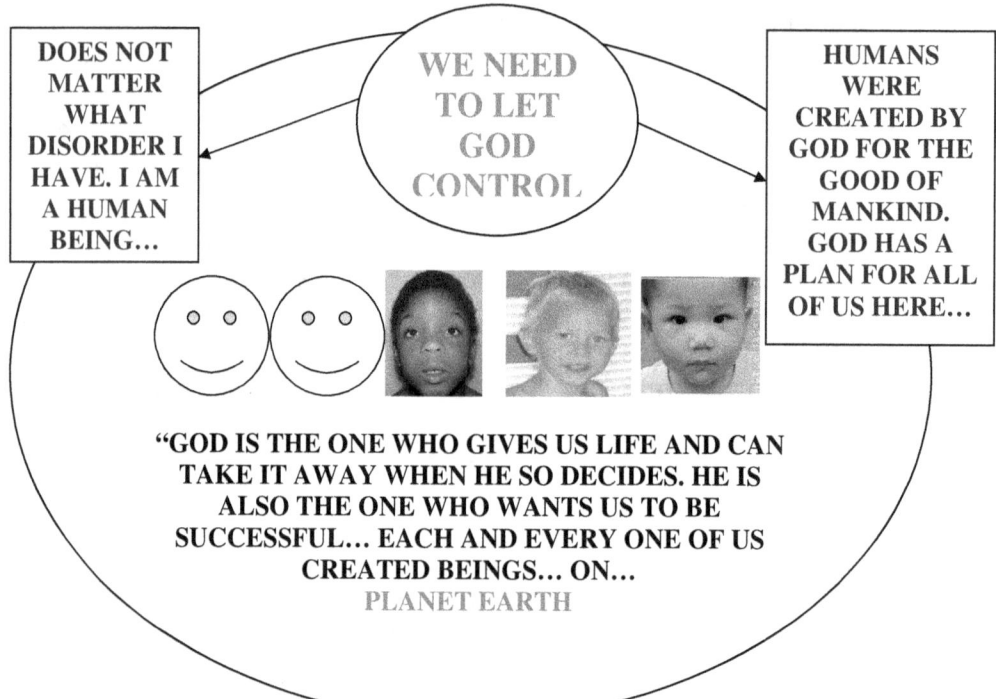

DOES NOT MATTER WHAT DISORDER I HAVE. I AM A HUMAN BEING...

WE NEED TO LET GOD CONTROL

HUMANS WERE CREATED BY GOD FOR THE GOOD OF MANKIND. GOD HAS A PLAN FOR ALL OF US HERE...

"GOD IS THE ONE WHO GIVES US LIFE AND CAN TAKE IT AWAY WHEN HE SO DECIDES. HE IS ALSO THE ONE WHO WANTS US TO BE SUCCESSFUL... EACH AND EVERY ONE OF US CREATED BEINGS... ON...
PLANET EARTH

SUMMARY:

You must have FAITH or life will be pointless. If you do not pursue your spirituality then you are living a life with a start point and an end point. We are created in the image of God. He has many images then. Each one is an offshoot of the real deal. It is said that humans are intelligent creatures... WE ARE ABLE TO FEEL... That makes us different. It takes effort to FEEL... It takes time to care... We have to stop and listen to be able to care... When we do that we grow and begin to understand. If we can do nothing to help, we may be able to in the future. Today take the time to listen and learn how to care just a little more.

It is the responsibility we have been given as human beings... THE RESPONSIBILITY TO CARE IS OUR GOD GIVEN DIRECTIVE... Find a situation in life to care about... One where you give without expecting anything in return...

"IT IS BETTER TO HAVE TRIED AND FAILED THAN NOT TO HAVE TRIED AT ALL. SUCCESS COMES TO THOSE WHO PERSEVERE"

By Henry Africa

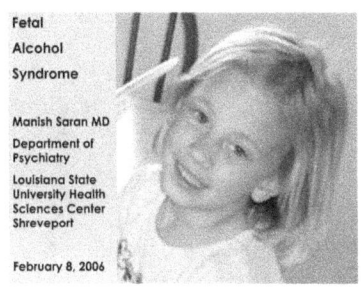

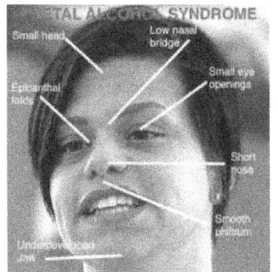

A SHOP… A CAR, A BUSINESS OR A HOLLIDAY OVERSEAS ARE ALL ATTAINABLE IF WE DEVELOP A FOCUSSED STRATEGY TO ACHIEVE THE GOAL. FAS CANNOT BE THE REASON THAT YOU DO NOT STRIVE TO ACHIEVE YOUR GOAL.

IT IS BY STRIVING THAT YOU ARE ALREADY A SUCCESS…

BY HENRY AFRICA

CHAPTER 4 FOUR

DID I MATTER SO LITTLE TO YOU THAT YOU DRANK

It is sometimes easy to get down on yourself when you are faced with societies intolerance to anyone who is different. As a person who has Fetal Alcohol Syndrome I face so much more challenges than people realize. Do they think life is easier for me because I may be deformed by this disorder? How can that make life easier for me? What about the reality we have to deal with every day? The reality that we had nothing to do with the way we look today? Do you stop for a minute before you judge and think about the consequence that face us because of what someone else has engineered. Someone who is normal looking and does not have to face societies judgmental attitude every time they walked into a shop or mall? There will never be a moment when my mother forgets that she made the mistake of drinking while she was pregnant. Will she take it out on me? Am I a reminder of the mistake she made by not abstaining from drinking during her pregnancy. Could she really care so little that she gave in to her habit, rather than fight for the right to have a perfectly normal child. I could have been if she had not drowned me in alcohol for 9 months…

SUMMARY:

Did you matter so little that your pregnant mother carried on drinking while she was pregnant with you? What do you know about what she went through during her pregnancy? Have you asked her why or is it above your emotional capacity to understand how to approach her regarding this issue? Do you keep the questions to yourself and beat yourself up about it whenever something happens to you? I would suggest that you ask her the questions that you have been asking yourself for so long. It will eat you up inside as long as you keep taking the blame for something you had no control over. Was your mother even aware of the dangers revolving around Fetal Alcohol Syndrome? Did she know the danger that drinking during pregnancy posed to her unborn child? Was she an addict who couldn't stop herself at the time and then quit after she was faced with the consequences of her actions? Could you forgive her if she had a reason that you could identify with? Is the fact that you hold this against her a way that you can cope with the consequences of her actions?... So many questions and so many answers that need to be found. But it will have to be faced if you are to remain sane and face all the other challenges that society will shovel in your direction. I use that phrase because it is the best one to describe having no power over what is going to come your way…

YOU MATTER TO GOD AND THAT IS THE ONLY PLACE TO GET COMFORT FROM…TRUST THAT GOD IS WITH YOU AND ASK THE QUESTIONS…

CHAPTER 5 FIVE

JOURNEY INSIDE MY HEAD – MY THOUGHTS

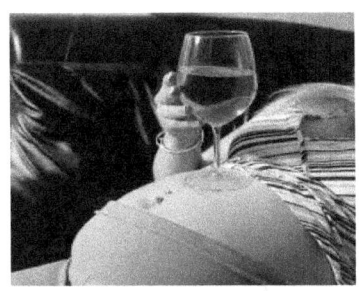

I cannot stop drinking wine. I have tried so many times but it is not very long then something happens and I literally run down to the bottle store to buy the next bottle of wine. My husband is hitting me. If I leave him now what will happen to my child. He got angry on the phone again just now. I bet he will want to hit me when he gets home tonight…

This stuff tonight tastes a little different than the milky stuff that comes down every day. Makes me light headed and then I laugh and kick for now reason. It's like a light starts flashing after I get a dose of this. The other milky stuff makes me sleepy. This makes me want to dance… Shake your boogy baby…

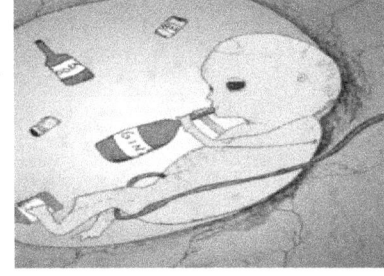

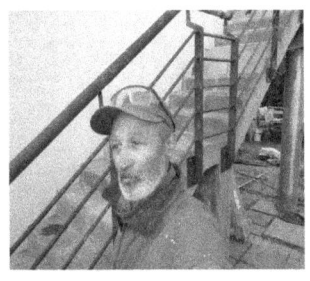

What thoughts go through an unborn child's mind when alcohol is induced into its body? The placenta carries whatever you are ingesting too. If you are giving your child the best then it will grow up and become a healthy baby. But if you drown it in 6.5ml of alcohol who knows what will come out of your womb when you give birth…

SUMMARY:

I am just saying things that may help you to work out in your head what you may be doing to yourself without thinking too hard. You can postpone those thought and then face the reality after 9 months or you can face the possible consequences now.

I THINK IT IS BETTER TO FACE THE CONSEQUENCES NOW. AND DO SOMETHING TO CHANGE THE POSSIBLE, DISASTEROUS CONSEQUENCES FROM BECOMING A REALITY…DON'T YOU?

BY HENRY AFRICA   **23**

"I AM THE SUM TOTAL OF THE EXPERIENCES THAT I AM ABLE TO ABSORB THROUGHOUT MY LIFE. IF I THINK I AM WORTH NOTHING THEN I ALLOW MYSELF TO BE WORTH NOTHING"

By Henry Africa

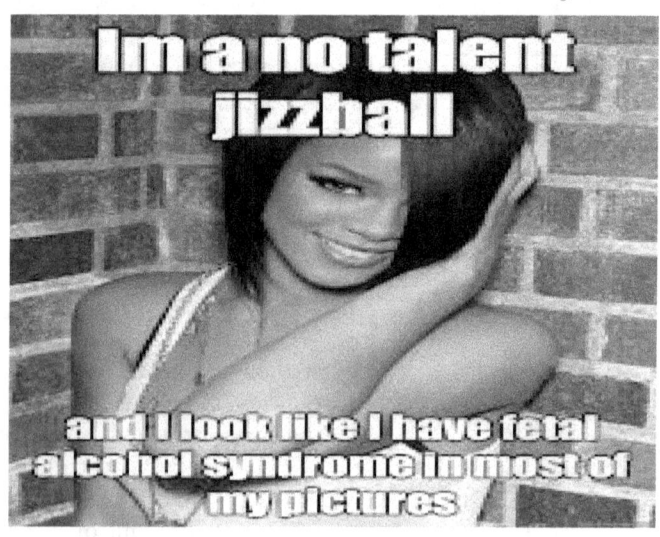

This is not a subject that deserves to be treated light-heartedly. The impact on people's lives is a grinding psychological battle that rages for every second that you are awake. The child needs to be monitored carefully every second of the day…

I hope that it is not something you take so lightly that you carry on **DRINKING ALCOHOL** when you are pregnant?

CHAPTER 5 FIVE

JOURNEY INSIDE MY HEAD – MY THOUGHTS

"Roslyn, how are you doing? It's been a while since we last spoke. You just disappeared and didn't bother to answer my calls," I said

"I was not in a good space Henry, Roslyn replied.

"What was the matter then? I said with concern.

"It's been something I have been thinking about for a long time. Should have told you…"

"Told me what Roslyn? We kind of drifted apart for no specific reason. I don't remember fighting with you about anything. We are still friends right?" I said.

"I was pregnant from you Henry. I decided not to tell you. I miscarried the child… There it was… Heart-breaking news that she had carried with her for a long time… What could I say? We were friends with benefits. It was at a time when we were both in need of a friend… One thing just led to another… For a while we were lovers. What could I say to her…Sorry I wasn't there for you? Wish you had told me? There was actually nothing I could say that would wipe the memory from her mind. She would always remember what happened. She had carried a life inside her for a while. What had caused the miscarriage? Her love of drinking and partying? We would never know for sure… A child that would have been born to two parents who had no intention of marrying? Think it was for the best… It was not an abortion by human hands maybe… God works for the good of all…Have to trust this was for the best… Neither of us decided to abort. I know I would not have told her to go for an abortion. I know she would not have gone for one…

SUMMARY:

This chapter deleted itself after I finished writing it. It was about something else when I wrote it the first time. Guess it reminds me how easy it would be to delete a fetus if it was found to be less than perfect in the womb. Just book an appointment and go for an abortion. Like pressing the delete button. But in this case you will do it with a full understanding of the murder you are going to commit. Can call it what you want but God sees it as murder. It's defined as the death of a human life…

Do you decide what is best in a case like this? Does God make mistakes? Is the end result of your drinking and drugs going to result in you committing murder to cover up for the original mistake you made? One mistake on top of another? Are you going to regret this act for the rest of your life too?

You will have to live with yourself after you walk out of the surgery rooms. You will wonder for the rest of your life if you made the right decision. And there is not a day that will go by that you will not remember what you did that day. Is the guilt worth living with?

WHO CAN TELL YOU WHAT THE RIGHT THING TO DO WOULD BE? I THINK I WOULD PRAY ABOUT IT AND TRUST GOD TO ADVISE ME…

BY HENRY AFRICA

CHAPTER 6 SIX

WE ARE BOTH VICTIMS NOW

"Miranda, I wish I had listened when my friends warned me against drinking alcohol during the time when I was pregnant. If I had listened then I may have had a perfectly healthy baby. Instead I have affected the future of my unborn child…"

"Shelley, I did not even know anything about this subject until I was 3 months pregnant. By then I must have been slamming back a bottle of Vodka a week. So loved the taste of Vodka and Orange juice. Guess my child was forced to drink it with me and it damaged his future…"

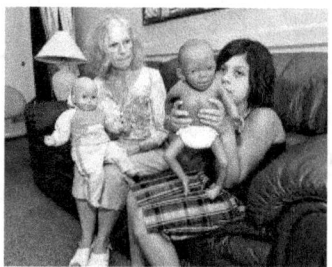

"I cannot take back the past Miranda. If I could then I would not go anywhere near alcohol during my pregnancy. Would not take even a glass of wine during that time. Next time I have a child I will make sure I do not drink alcohol at all…"

Shelley, I do not even feel like I want to ever be pregnant again. What if this happens again? What if something new affects me during the pregnancy/ I cannot imagine having 2 children with some birth deformity or other…

SUMMARY

Yes, that is the reality in this story. The child suffered because of the behavior of the parent. You are both victims now. If you carry on beating yourself over the head then nothing positive will evolve in your future. You have to love that child and be strong for that child. You have to forgive yourself even though you will have to face the extent of your mistake every day for 365 days a year. The child may never leave home as a normal child will. Challenges are immense for them. You have to bury your guilt and draw closer to God. Only God can rid you of this guilt. If you do not then you are no good to the future of your child… Your child still needs you to be courageous…

YOU MUST FORGIVE YOURSELF… GOD FORGIVES YOU…

BY HENRY AFRICA   **26**

"ONE DAY DOES NOT DEFINE A MAN OR WOMAN. WE ALL HAVE THE ABILITY TO CREATE OUR OWN LEGACY."

QUOTE FROM THE MOVIE MISSION PARK

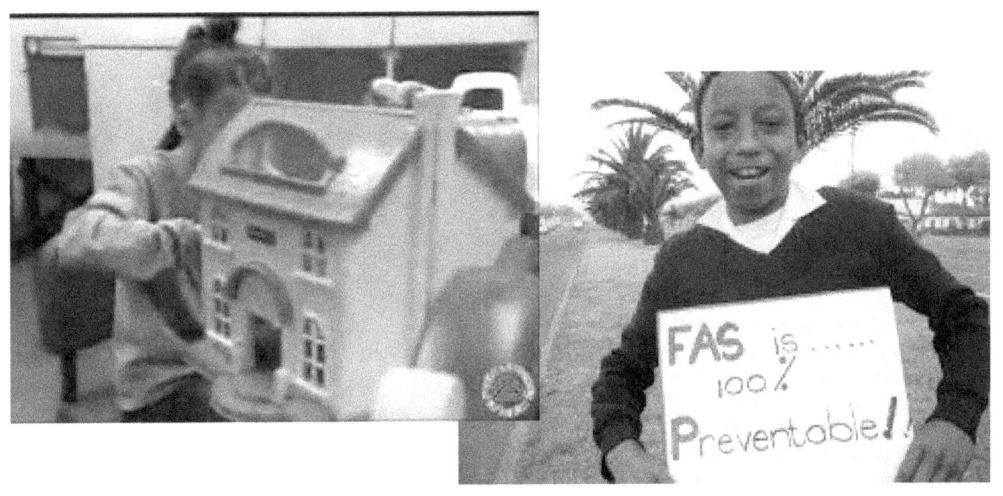

IT MAY BE DIFFICULT BUT YOU CAN DO IT IF YOU JUST BELIEVE IN YOURSELF AND ACCEPT THE ROLE YOU HAVE BEEN CAST IN.

DON'T LET NEGATIVE EMOTIONS OVERWELM YOU AS YOU STRIVE TO E A SUCCESS. SOME THINGS CANNOT BE CHANGED. ACCEPTANCE IS THE FIRST STEP TOWARDS YOUR LIFE SUCCESS...

WHAT IS DONE IS DONE... ACCEPT THAT AND MOVE ON...

BY HENRY AFRICA

CHAPTER 6 SIX

WE ARE BOTH VICTIMS NOW

"Timothy, what are you doing here? I asked him as I stood looking at my old friend…
"I am attending the Alcoholics Anonymous Meeting in that room," He added.
"You have an alcohol problem? I said dumbfounded
"Yes," he said… "Have had this problem for a while and it's combined with drugs too"
"That is hard for me to believe Tim," I said… "You look like you got it all together"
"Yes Henry! That may be the way it looks to people from the outside looking in"

That conversation was real. It took place at a public school where someone had decided to do something about the pain a particular group of people where suffering through. Sadly Timothy is no longer with us today. He succumbed to his addiction or the side effects of them. He lost the battle to live. He died before he was destined to. A sad loss to all the friends who knew him.

SUMMARY

Timothy was a famous rugby player who rose to the top in the sport here in our local community. Many people knew about his struggles with alcohol. I was one of the last people to find out about the struggles he had been facing. I knew that he had experimented with drugs at an early age. Somehow I did not follow the tragic path that led to his early death from a drug habit that systematically destroyed his body.

The body cannot take constant punishment from drugs and harmful toxins. It has mechanisms to clean itself out but how many times can we punish our bodies without having some kind of organ failure occur. But is it that easy to conquer the addiction? Drugs, substances can addict us after a single use today. It does not take our bodies long to get addicted to alcohol. One drink can establish a habit that can lead to an addiction. With drugs one use can lead to instant addiction. Some people are more obsessive compulsive than others. They will connect the dots and enjoy the experience the first time and want repeats on a regular basis. The road is a downhill one… It is best not to even try drugs once. Especially the highly addictive and toxic drugs they have on the market today. Given it is a black market. In this case black means possible death by substance abuse over the years thereafter. You can conquer the addiction but it will take you a while. Rehabilitation does not take place overnight. The temptation will always be there…

BE PREAPRED FOR A RELAPSE OR TWO. It will not be easy but it will be worthwhile to conquer that addiction… Keep on trying and persevere till you do…

CHAPTER *7* SEVEN
WHAT HAS THE PAST DONE TO ME

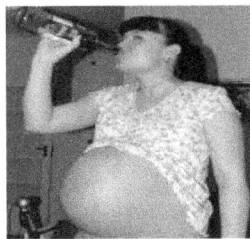

They say old habits die hard. It may be a saying to most people but it is really a truth to me. I wish I didn't have this habit because with my pregnancy I have found it the hardest habit to get rid of.

Who in their right mind would risk the health of their unborn child if they had a choice? I am in a struggle to give up this habit. Help me don't judge me…

"I am having supper with you tonight Mom. Then we will have breakfast together and maybe lunch too. For the next 9 months you are going to share every meal that you have with me. I am your date for the next 9 months. Dont do what your mother did…

Try and get us some really nice things to eat ok? Please try your best mom?"

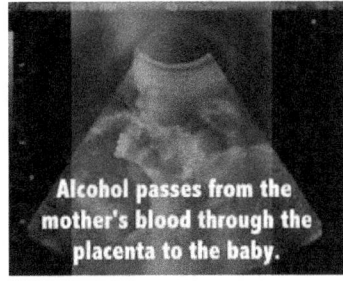

Alcohol passes from the mother's blood through the placenta to the baby.

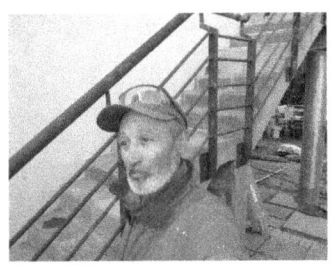

In the past you ate and drank just what you pleased. Now that you are pregnant with a child, you need to watch what you are going to eat. It is a choice that will make the difference between having a healthy child or maybe not. Give your child the best chance of being born healthy by not drinking Alcohol during your pregnancy. It's the least you can do…

SUMMARY:

Maybe economic times are hard for you. Maybe you are unemployed and have to struggle to provide for your unborn child. But trust and believe that God will provide for his child. It is not entirely your child. Even if the natural father does not do so then you can get help from some other source. The one thing that will make you sure of having a healthy child is to avoid alcohol during your pregnancy. Alcohol and drugs will be carried via the bloodstream to your unborn child. The past does not rule what you do whilst pregnant…

BY HENRY AFRICA **29**

"EVERYTHING IN LIFE IS EITHER GROWING OR DYING. IF YOU ARE NOT BUSY HELPING TO BUILD UP THEN YOU ARE BUSY HELPING TO BREAK DOWN..."

By Henry Africa

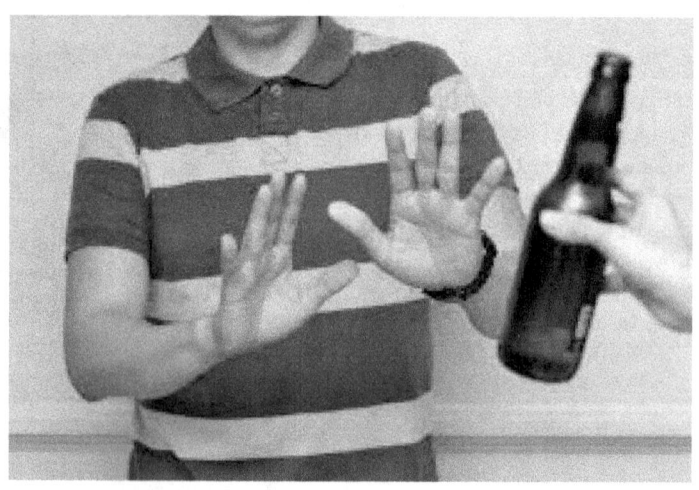

LIFE IS FILLED WITH CHOICES. EVERYONE DOES NOT DRINK ALCOHOL... EVERYONE DOES NOT SMOKE CIGARETTES OR DO DRUGS... EVERYONE DOES NOT DO SEX BEFORE MARRIAGE...

CHOOSE THE GROUP OF FRIENDS WHO YOU WILL GROW UP WITH AND FOLLOW THE GOOD SET OF VALUES THAT THEY WILL HELP YOU TO BE A PART OF. DON'T LET THE NEED FOR FRIENDS MAKE YOU CHOOSE THE WRONG ONES. THE RIGHT FRIENDS WILL COME ALONG AS YOU MATURE AND FIND YOUR PLACE IN THIS WORLD... THERE IS A PLACE FOR ALL OF US... WE NEED TO TRUST GOD AND BE PATIENT...

CHAPTER 7 SEVEN

WHAT HAS THE PAST DONE TO ME

I have been raised knowing all the time that I should not drink during my pregnancy. I didn't know I would be having a baby at the time I am suffering from depression. Drinking helps me to overcome the emotions relating to the depression. The thoughts of suicide are driven away when I have a few drinks and then life seems easier to bear. Now that I am pregnant I have tried to go without the alcohol but have experienced such devastating feelings that I felt like jumping off the 20th floor of the tallest building in town. I hate myself when I feel like that but the medication does help and the alcohol too. At times like this…

I have been living since birth with parents who drink and do drugs. The social welfare people took me away from them and placed me in one foster home after the other. No one really wanted me. As long as they received a grant they were prepared to keep me. Then they found out how difficult it was to raise a child with FETAL ALCOHOL SYNDROME. Very soon they would find a reason to return me to the social services and then it was back to an orphanage. I was angry a lot of the time. Was neglected and had to live in so many different homes that I never got to make any friends I can remember. Was this my fault? How did the past affect the future that I faced? I don't see my parents anymore. They do not even look for me. Hear they have another child... A healthy one… How could they do that to me…?

SUMMARY

It was my mother's drinking and substance abuse that led to me being what I am. I may be a slow learner and that leads to impatience on people's part. They start out being patient but lose that patience after having to repeat themselves over and over again. I cannot remember what they said last week. It is not my fault I am told. My mother gave birth normally and there were no complications. The doctors said that the deformities I suffered were due to her drinking excessively during the time she was pregnant. She has unknowingly given me the worst gift possible. She has created a deformed version of who I could have been. She may as well have designed me by the lifestyle she chose. I am prone to violence. I am told this is normal. They tell me 90% of FAS sufferers have mental health problems... 80% have trouble holding onto a job and most lack impulse control. I never chose to have those problems but it is my destiny now. 6-0% of us will end up behind bars at some stage of our lives. Don't quite understand how? Due to losing tempers and of property destruction? End up in treatment centers over lifespan… In drugs and alcohol due to condition? Had my 1st drink before I was born…

HOW IS IT POSSIBLE THAT SOMEONE WOULD TRY AND HAVE A CHILD KNOWING THE KINDS OF RISKS THEIR BEEHAVIOR POSED. Perhaps I would have been better off if they had aborted me…

CHAPTER 8 EIGHT

WHAT HAVE I MISSED

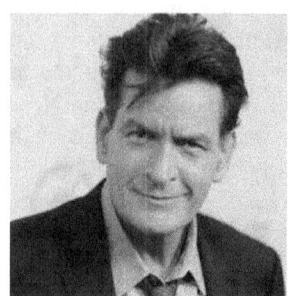

Can I be a movie Star? Could I become a famous politician? Could I be a top sports star? Will I be able to walk on the red carpet at the Academy Awards one day?

YES!! Everything is possible to those who have a little FAITH... Faith like a mustard seed... That is what Jesus Christ said. God believes we can overcome anything... Who are we to argue...?

My friend Graham Roodt surveyed the damage and told me afterwards how the accident happened. The people have either died or been badly injured in this accident... Someone has brain damage too. That is tragic...

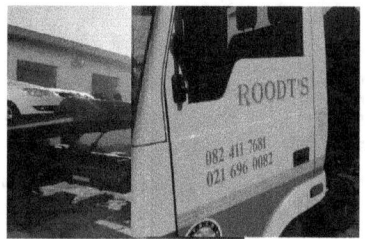

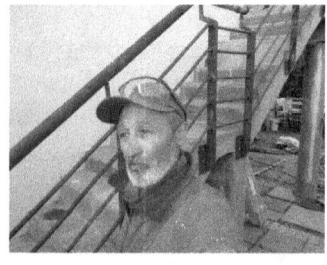

If you have Fetal Alcohol Syndrome then you must fight to overcome the challenges you will face. You do not have a mental condition that condemns you to a life of lesser quality.

Suffering brain damage may be a bit more serious. Or is there any difference? Can either challenge be easier? **NO!!** Just do your best...

SUMMARY:

We have to try and help others as we progress through life. There are many times we may be able to make a positive difference to the lives of others. My friend graham is worth mentioning here. He is going to be unhappy that I am talking about this. He donates money from his business to worthy causes on an annual basis... HE IS A GREAT EXAMPLE TO HIS FAMILY AND ALSO TO HIS FRIENDS.

AN EXAMPLE WORTH IMITATING...YOU BE THAT WAY TOO

"A WISE MAN LEARNS BY HIS MISTAKES. A WISER MAN WILL LEARN BY THE MISTAKES OF OTHERS"

By Mark Sanchez

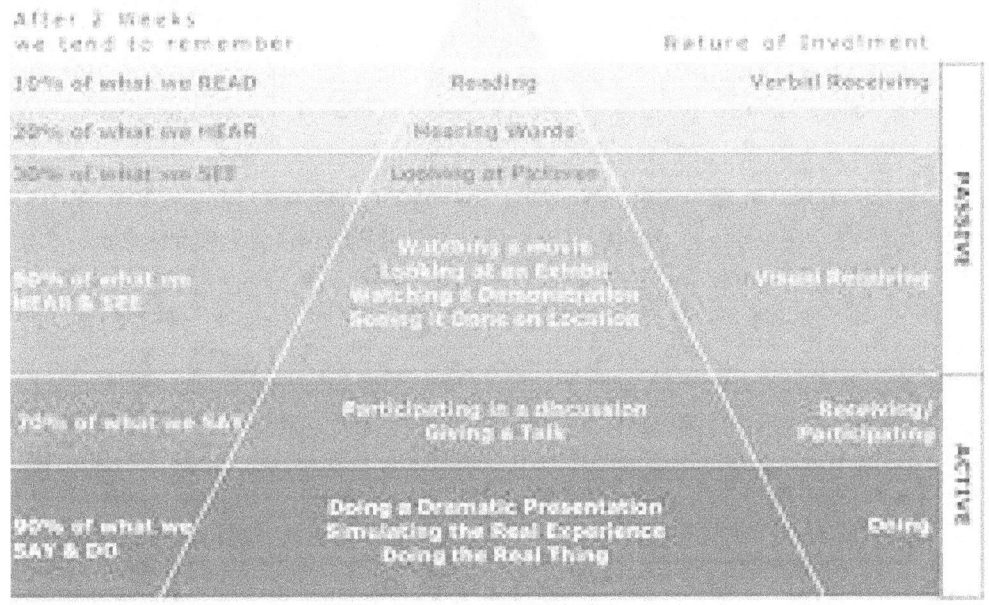

WE ALL WILL MAKE MISTAKES. BE A WISE PERSON AND DO NOT REPEAT THE MISTAKES YOU MAKE TODAY...

CHAPTER 8 EIGHT

WHAT HAVE I MISSED

Fetal alcohol syndrome – Ex Wikipedia sources

FULL CREDIT FOR INFORMATION SUPPLIED GOES TO UNKNOWNWIKIPEDIA SUPPLY SOURCES

Fetal alcohol syndrome (FAS) or foetal alcohol syndrome (see spelling differences) is a pattern of mental and physical defects that can develop in a fetus in association with high levels of alcohol consumption during pregnancy. Alcohol crosses the placental barrier and can stunt fetal growth or weight, create distinctive facial stigmata, damage neurons and brain structures, which can result in psychological or behavioral problems, and cause other physical damage. The main effect of FAS is permanent central nervous system damage, especially to the brain. Developing brain cells and structures can be malformed or have development interrupted by prenatal alcohol exposure; this can create an array of primary cognitive and functional disabilities (including poor memory, attention deficits, impulsive behavior, and poor cause-effect reasoning) as well as secondary disabilities (for example, predispositions to mental health problems and drug addiction). Alcohol exposure presents a risk of fetal brain damage at any point during a pregnancy, since brain development is ongoing throughout pregnancy.

As of 1987, fetal alcohol exposure was the leading known cause of intellectual disability in the Western world.[1] In the United States and Europe, the FAS prevalence rate is estimated to be between 0.2–2 in every 1000 live births. FAS should not be confused with Fetal Alcohol Spectrum Disorders (FASD), a condition which describes a continuum of permanent birth defects caused by maternal consumption of alcohol during pregnancy, which includes FAS, as well as other disorders, and which affects about 1% of live births in the US (i.e., about 10 cases per 1000 live births). The lifetime medical and social costs of FAS are estimated to be as high as US$800,000 per child born with the disorder. Surveys found that in the United States, 10–15% of pregnant women report having recently drunk alcohol, and up to 30% drink alcohol at some point during pregnancy. The current recommendation of the Surgeon General of the United States, the British Department of Health and the Australian Government National Health and Medical Research Council is to drink no alcohol at all during pregnancy.

Growth Deficiency

Growth deficiency is defined as below average height, weight or both due to prenatal alcohol exposure, and can be assessed at any point in the lifespan. Growth measurements must be adjusted for parental height, gestational age(for a premature infant), and other postnatal insults (e.g., poor nutrition), although birth height and weight are the preferred measurements. Deficiencies are documented H191 when height or weight falls at or below the 10th percentile of standardized growth charts appropriate to the patient's population.

The CDC and Canadian guidelines use the 10th percentile as a cut-off to determine growth deficiency The "4-Digit Diagnostic Code" (4-DDC), allows for mid-range gradations in growth deficiency (between the 3rd and 10th percentiles) and severe growth deficiency at or below the 3rd percentile.[11] Growth deficiency (at severe, moderate, or mild levels) contributes to diagnoses of FAS and PFAS (Partial Fetal Alcohol Syndrome), but not ARND (Alcohol-Related Neurodevelopment Disorder) or static encephalopathy.

Growth deficiency is ranked as follows by the 4-DDC.

- Severe — Height and weight at or below the 3rd percentile.

- Moderate — Either height or weight at or below the 3rd percentile, but not both.

- Mild — Both height and weight between the 3rd and 10th percentiles.

- None — Height and weight both above the 10th percentile.

Facial features

Several characteristic craniofacial abnormalities are often visible in individuals with FAS.[24] The presence of FAS facial features indicates brain damage, though brain damage may also exist in their absence. FAS facial features (and most other visible, but non-diagnostic, deformities) are believed to be caused mainly during the 10th and 20th week of gestation.

Refinements in diagnostic criteria since 1975 have yielded three distinctive and diagnostically significant facial features known to result from prenatal alcohol exposure and distinguishes FAS from other disorders with partially overlapping characteristics. The three FAS facial features are:

- A smooth philtrum — The divot or groove between the nose and upper lip flattens with increased prenatal alcohol exposure.

- Thin vermilion — The upper lip thins with increased prenatal alcohol exposure.

- Small palpebral fissures — Eye width decreases with increased prenatal alcohol exposure.

Measurement of FAS facial features uses criteria developed by the University of Washington. The lip and philtrum are measured by a trained physician with the Lip-Philtrum Guide, a 5-point Likert Scale with representative photographs of lip and philtrum combinations ranging from normal (ranked 1) to severe (ranked 5). Palpebral fissure length (PFL) is measured in millimeters with either calipers or a clear ruler and then compared to a PFL growth chart, also developed by the University of Washington.

Ranking FAS facial features is complicated because the three separate facial features can be affected independently by prenatal alcohol. A summary of the criteria follows

- Severe — All three facial features ranked independently as severe (lip ranked at 4 or 5, philtrum ranked at 4 or 5, and PFL two or more standard deviations below average).

- Moderate — Two facial features ranked as severe and one feature ranked as moderate (lip *or* philtrum ranked at 3, *or* PFL between one and two standard deviations below average).

- Mild — A mild ranking of FAS facial features covers a broad range of facial feature combinations:

  - Two facial features ranked severe and one ranked within normal limits,

  - One facial feature ranked severe and two ranked moderate, or

  - One facial feature ranked severe, one ranked moderate and one ranked within normal limits.

- None — All three facial features ranked within normal limits.

These distinctive facial features in a patient do strongly correlate to brain damage. Sterling Clarren of the University of Washington's Fetal Alcohol and Drug Unit told a conference in 2002:

"I have never seen anybody with this whole face who doesn't have some brain damage. In fact in studies, as the face is more FAS-like, the brain is more likely to be abnormal. The only face that you would want to counsel people or predict the future about is the full FAS face. But the risk of brain damage increases as the eyes get smaller, as the philtrum gets flatter, and the lip gets thinner. The risk goes up but not the diagnosis."

"At one-month gestation, the top end of your body is a brain, and at the very front end of that early brain, there is tissue that has been brain tissue. It stops being brain and gets ready to be your face ... Your eyeball is also brain tissue. It's an extension of the second part of the brain. It started as brain and "popped out." So if you are going to look at parts of the brain from alcohol damage, or any kind of damage during pregnancy, eye malformations and midline facial malformations are going to be very actively related to the brain across syndromes ... and they certainly are with FAS.

Central nervous system

Central nervous system (CNS) damage is the primary feature of any Fetal Alcohol Spectrum Disorder (FASD) diagnosis. Prenatal exposure to alcohol — which is classified as teratogen — can damage the brain across a continuum of gross to subtle impairments, depending on the amount, timing, and frequency of the exposure as well as genetic predispositions of the fetus and mother. While functional abnormalities are the behavioral and cognitive expressions of the FAS disability, CNS damage can be assessed in three areas: structural, neurological, and functional impairments.

All four diagnostic systems allow for assessment of CNS damage in these areas, but criteria vary. The IOM system requires structural or neurological impairment for a diagnosis of FAS.[19] The 4-DDC and CDC guidelines state that functional anomalies must measure at two standard deviations or worse in three or more functional domains for a diagnosis of FAS. The 4-DDC further elaborates the degree of CNS damage according to four ranks:

• Definite — Structural impairments or neurological impairments for FAS or static encephalopathy.

• Probable — Significant dysfunction of two standard deviations or worse in three or more functional domains.

• Possible — Mild to moderate dysfunction of two standard deviations or worse in one or two functional domains *or* by judgment of the clinical evaluation team that CNS damage cannot be dismissed.

• Unlikely — No evidence of CNS damage.

Structural

Structural abnormalities of the brain are observable, physical damage to the brain or brain structures caused by prenatal alcohol exposure. Structural impairments may include microcephaly (small head size) of two or more standard deviations below the average, or other abnormalities in brain structure (e.g., agenesis of the corpus callosum, cerebellar hypoplasia).

Microcephaly is determined by comparing head circumference (often called occipito frontal circumference, or OFC) to appropriate OFC growth charts. Other structural impairments must be observed through medical imaging techniques by a trained physician. Because imaging procedures are expensive and relatively inaccessible to most patients, diagnosis of FAS is not frequently made via structural impairments, except for microcephaly.

Evidence of a CNS structural impairment due to prenatal alcohol exposure will result in a diagnosis of FAS, and neurological and functional impairments are highly likely.

During the first trimester of pregnancy, alcohol interferes with the migration and organization of brain cells, which can create structural deformities or deficits within the brain. During the third trimester, damage can be caused to the hippocampus, which plays a role in memory, learning, emotion, and encoding visual and auditory information, all of which can create neurological and functional CNS impairments as well.

As of 2002, there were 25 reports of autopsies on infants known to have FAS. The first was in 1973, on an infant who died shortly after birth. The examination revealed extensive brain damage, including microcephaly, migration anomalies, callosal dysgenesis, and a massive neuroglial, leptomeningeal heterotopia covering the left hemisphere.

In 1977, Dr. Clarren described a second infant whose mother was a binge drinker. The infant died ten days after birth. The autopsy showed severe hydrocephalus, abnormal neuronal migration, and a small corpus callosum (which connects the two brain hemispheres) and cerebellum. FAS has also been linked to brainstem and cerebellar changes, agenesis of the corpus callosum and anterior commissure, neuronal migration errors, absent olfactory bulbs, meningomyelocele, and porencephaly.

Neurological

When structural impairments are not observable or do not exist, neurological impairments are assessed. In the context of FAS, neurological impairments are caused by prenatal alcohol exposure which causes general neurological damage to the central nervous system (CNS) and the peripheral nervous system (PNS). A determination of a neurological problem must be made by a trained physician, and must not be due to a postnatal insult, such as a high fever, concussion, traumatic brain injury, etc.

All four diagnostic systems show virtual agreement on their criteria for CNS damage at the neurological level, and evidence of a CNS neurological impairment due to prenatal alcohol exposure will result in a diagnosis of FAS, and functional impairments are highly likely.

Neurological problems are expressed as either hard signs, or diagnosable disorders, such as epilepsy or other seizure disorders, or soft signs. Soft signs are broader, nonspecific neurological impairments, or symptoms, such as impaired fine motor skills, neurosensory hearing loss, poor gait, clumsiness, poor eye-hand coordination. Many soft signs have normal-referenced criteria, while others are determined through clinical judgment. "Clinical judgment" is only as good as the clinician, and soft signs should be assessed by either a pediatric neurologist, a pediatric neuropsychologist, or both. Those affected have mild retardation.

Functional

When structural or neurological impairments are not observed, all four diagnostic systems allow CNS damage due to prenatal alcohol exposure to be assessed in terms of functional impairments. Functional impairments are deficits, problems, delays, or abnormalities due to prenatal alcohol exposure (rather than hereditary causes or postnatal insults) in observable and measurable domains related to daily functioning, often referred to as developmental disabilities. There is no consensus on a specific pattern of functional impairments due to prenatal alcohol exposure—and only CDC guidelines label developmental delays as such, so criteria vary somewhat across diagnostic systems.

The four diagnostic systems list various CNS domains that can qualify for functional impairment that can determine an FAS diagnosis:

- Evidence of a complex pattern of behavior or cognitive abnormalities inconsistent with developmental level in the following CNS domains — sufficient for a PFAS (partial fetal alcohol syndrome) or ARND (alcohol-related neurodevelopmental disorder) diagnosis using IOM guidelines

    - Learning disabilities, academic achievement, impulse control, social perception, communication, abstraction, math skills, memory, attention, judgment

- Performance at two or more standard deviations on standardized testing in three or more of the following CNS domains — sufficient for a FAS, PFAS or static encephalopathy diagnosis using the 4-DDC.[11]

    - Executive functioning, memory, cognition, social/adaptive skills, academic achievement, language, motor skills, attention, activity level

- General cognitive deficits (e.g., IQ) at or below the 3rd percentile on standardized testing — sufficient for an FAS diagnosis using CDC guidelines

➤ Performance at or below the 16th percentile on standardized testing in three or more of the following CNS domains — sufficient for an FAS diagnosis using CDC guidelines

    ➤ Cognition, executive functioning, motor functioning, attention and hyperactive problems, social skills, sensory processing disorder, social communication, memory, difficulties responding to common parenting practices

➤ Performance at two or more standard deviations on standardized testing in three or more of the following CNS domains — sufficient for an FAS diagnosis using Canadian guidelines

    ➤ Cognition, communication, academic achievement, memory, executive functioning, adaptive behavior, social skills, social communication

Related signs

Other conditions may commonly co-occur with FAS, stemming from prenatal alcohol exposure. However, these conditions are considered Alcohol-Related Birth Defects and not diagnostic criteria for FAS.

➤ Cardiac — A heart murmur that frequently disappears by one year of age. Ventricular septal defect most commonly seen, followed by an atrial septal defect.

➤ Skeletal — Joint anomalies including abnormal position and function, altered palmar crease patterns, small distal phalanges, and small fifth fingernails.

➤ Renal — Horseshoe, aplastic, dysplastic, or hypo plastic kidneys.

➤ Ocular — Strabismus, optic nerve hypoplasia (which may cause light sensitivity, decreased visual acuity, or involuntary eye movements).

➤ Occasional abnormalities — ptosis of the eyelid, micro-ophthalmia, cleft lip with or without a cleft palate, webbed neck, short neck, tetralogy of Fallot, coarctation of the aorta, spina bifida, and hydrocephalus.

Cause

Prenatal alcohol exposure is the cause of fetal alcohol syndrome. A study of over 400,000 American women, all of whom had consumed alcohol during pregnancy, concluded that consumption of 15 drinks or more per week was associated with a reduction in birth weight. Though consumption of less than 15 drinks per week was not proven to cause FAS-related effects, the study authors recommend limiting consumption to no more than one standard drink per day. Also, threshold values are based upon group averages, and it is not appropriate to conclude that exposure below this threshold is necessarily 'safe' because of the significant individual variations in alcohol pharmacokinetics. An analysis of seven medical research studies involving over 130,000 pregnancies found that consuming two to 14 drinks per week did not significantly increase the risk of giving birth to a child with either malformations or fetal alcohol syndrome.[39] Pregnant women who consume approximately 144 grams of pure alcohol per day have a 30–33% chance of having a baby with FAS.

A number of studies have shown that light drinking (1–2 drinks/week) during pregnancy does not appear to pose a risk to the fetus A study of pregnancies in eight European countries found that consuming no more than one drink per day did not appear to have any effect on fetal growth. A follow-up of children at 18 months of age found that those from women who drank during pregnancy, even two drinks per day, scored higher in several areas of development, though in a different study, as little as one drink per day resulted in poorer spelling and reading abilities at age 6 and a linear dose-response relationship was seen between prenatal alcohol exposure and poorer arithmetic scores at the same age.

Biochemical pathways

Despite intense research efforts, it has not been possible to identify a single clear-cut mechanism for development of FAS or FASD. On the contrary, clinical and animal studies have identified a broad spectrum of pathways through which maternal alcohol can negatively affect the outcome of a pregnancy. Clear conclusions with universal validity are difficult to draw, since different ethnic groups show considerable genetic polymorphism for the hepatic enzymes responsible for ethanol detoxification

A human fetus appears to be at triple risk from maternal alcohol consumption:

1. The placenta allows free entry of ethanol and toxic metabolites like acetaldehyde into the fetal compartment. The so-called placental barrier is no barrier with respect to ethanol.

2. The developing fetal nervous system appears particularly sensitive to ethanol toxicity. The latter impacts negatively on proliferation, differentiation, neuronal migration, axonic outgrowth, integration and fine tuning of the synaptic network. In short, all major processes in the developing central nervous system appear compromised.

3. Fetal tissues are quite different from adult tissues in function and purpose. For example, the main detoxicating organ in adults is the liver, whereas fetal liver is

incapable of detoxicating ethanol as the ADH and ALDH enzymes have not yet been brought to expression at this early stage. Up to term, fetal tissues do not have significant capacity for the detoxification of ethanol, and the fetus remains exposed to ethanol in the amniotic fluid for periods far longer than the decay time of ethanol in the maternal circulation.

Generally, fetal tissues have far less antioxidant protection than adult tissues as they express no significant quantities ADH or ALDH, and far less antioxidant enzymes like SOD, glutathion transferases or glutathion peroxidases

Diagnosis

Several diagnostic systems have been developed in North America:

> - The Institute of Medicine's guidelines for FAS, the first system to standardize diagnoses of individuals with prenatal alcohol exposure,

> - The University of Washington's 4-DDC, which ranks the four key features of FASD on a Likert scale of one to four and yields 256 descriptive codes that can be categorized into 22 distinct clinical categories, ranging from FAS to no findings

> - The Centers for Disease Control's "Fetal Alcohol Syndrome: Guidelines for Referral and Diagnosis," which established general consensus on the diagnosis FAS in the U.S. but deferred addressing other FASD conditions, and

> - Canadian guidelines for FASD diagnosis, which established criteria for diagnosing FASD in Canada and harmonized most differences between the IOM and University of Washington's systems.

Fetal alcohol syndrome is the only expression of FASD that has garnered consensus among experts to become an official ICD-9 and ICD-10 diagnosis. To make this diagnosis (or determine any FASD condition), a multi-disciplinary evaluation is necessary to assess each of the four key features for assessment. Generally, a trained physician will determine growth deficiency and FAS facial features. While a qualified physician may also assess central nervous system structural abnormalities and/or neurological problems, usually central nervous system damage is determined through psychological assessment. A pediatric neuropsychologist may assess all areas of functioning, including intellectual, language processing, and sensorimotor. Prenatal alcohol exposure risk may be assessed by a qualified physician or psychologist.

The following criteria must be fully met for an FAS diagnosis.

1. Growth deficiency — Prenatal or postnatal height or weight (or both) at or below the 10th percentile

2. FAS facial features — All three FAS facial features present

3. Central nervous system damage — Clinically significant structural, neurological, *or* functional impairment

4. Prenatal alcohol exposure — Confirmed or Unknown prenatal alcohol exposure

Alcohol intake is determined by interview of the biological mother or other family members knowledgeable of the mother's alcohol use during the pregnancy, prenatal health records, and review of available birth records, court records, chemical dependency treatment records, or other reliable sources. Exposure level is assessed as Confirmed Exposure, Unknown Exposure, and Confirmed Absence of Exposure by the IOM, CDC and Canadian diagnostic systems. The 4-DDC further distinguishes confirmed exposure as High Risk and Some Risk:

➢ High Risk — Confirmed use of alcohol during pregnancy known to be at high blood alcohol levels (100 mg/dL or greater) delivered at least weekly in early pregnancy.

➢ Some Risk — Confirmed use of alcohol during pregnancy with use less than High Risk or unknown usage patterns.

➢ Unknown Risk — Unknown use of alcohol during pregnancy.

➢ No Risk — Confirmed absence of prenatal alcohol exposure, which rules out an FAS diagnosis.

Confirmed exposure

Amount, frequency, and timing of prenatal alcohol use can dramatically impact the other three key features of FAS. While consensus exists that alcohol is a teratogen, there is no clear consensus as to what level of exposure is toxic. The CDC guidelines are silent on these elements diagnostically. The IOM and Canadian guidelines explore this further, acknowledging the importance of significant alcohol exposure from regular or heavy episodic alcohol consumption in determining, but offer no standard for diagnosis. Canadian guidelines discuss this lack of clarity and parenthetically point out that "heavy alcohol use" is defined by the National Institute on Alcohol Abuse and Alcoholism as five or more drinks per episode on five or more days during a 30 day period.

The 4-DDC ranking system distinguishes between levels of prenatal alcohol exposure as *High Risk* and *Some Risk*. It operationalizes high risk exposure as a blood alcohol concentration (BAC) greater than 100 mg/dL delivered at least weekly in early pregnancy. This BAC level is typically reached by a 55 kg woman drinking six to eight beers in one sitting.

Unknown exposure

For many adopted or adult patients and children in foster care, records or other reliable sources may not be available for review. Reporting alcohol use during pregnancy can also be stigmatizing to birth mothers, especially if alcohol use is ongoing.[22] In these cases, all diagnostic systems use an unknown prenatal alcohol exposure designation. A diagnosis of FAS is still possible with an unknown exposure level if other key features of FASD are present at clinical levels.

Differential diagnosis

The CDC reviewed nine syndromes that have overlapping features with FAS; however, none of these syndromes include all three FAS facial features, and none are the result of prenatal alcohol exposure.

- Aarskog syndrome
- Williams syndrome
- Noonan syndrome
- Dubowitz syndrome
- Brachman-DeLange syndrome
- Toluene syndrome
- Fetal hydantoin syndrome
- Fetal valproate syndrome
- Maternal PKU fetal effects

Prevention

The only certain way to prevent FAS is to simply avoid drinking alcohol during pregnancy. In the United States, the Surgeon General recommended in 1981, and again in 2005, that women abstain from alcohol use while pregnant or while planning a pregnancy, the latter to avoid damage in the earliest stages of a pregnancy, as the woman may not be aware that she has conceived. In the United States, federal legislation has required that warning labels be placed on all alcoholic beverage containers since 1988 under the Alcoholic Beverage Labeling Act.

Treatment

There is no cure for FAS, because the CNS damage creates a permanent disability, but treatment is possible. Because CNS damage, symptoms, secondary disabilities, and needs vary widely by individual, there is no one treatment type that works for everyone.

Medical interventions

Traditional medical interventions (i.e., psychoactive drugs) are frequently tried on those with FAS because many FAS symptoms are mistaken for or overlap with other disorders, most notably ADHD.[50]

Behavioral interventions

Traditional behavioral interventions are predicated on learning theory, which is the basis for many parenting and professional strategies and interventions.[51] Along with ordinary parenting styles, such strategies are frequently used by default for treating those with FAS, as the diagnoses Oppositional Defiance Disorder (ODD), Conduct Disorder, Reactive Attachment Disorder (RAD), etc. often overlap with FAS (along with ADHD), and these are sometimes thought to benefit from behavioral interventions. Frequently, a patient's poor academic achievement results in special education services, which also utilizes principles of learning theory, behavior modification, and outcome-based education.

Because the "learning system" of a patient with FAS is damaged, however, behavioral interventions are not always successful, or not successful in the long run, especially because overlapping disorders frequently stem from or are exacerbated by FAS.[51] Kohn (1999) suggests that a rewards-punishment system in general may work somewhat in the short term but is unsuccessful in the long term because that approach fails to consider content (i.e., things "worth" learning), community (i.e., safe, cooperative learning environments), and choice (i.e., making choices versus following directions).[52] While these elements are important to consider when working with FAS and have some usefulness in treatment, they are not alone sufficient to promote better outcomes.[51] Kohn's minority challenge to behavioral interventions does illustrate the importance of factors beyond learning theory when trying to promote improved outcomes for FAS, and supports a more multi-model approach that can be found in varying degrees within the advocacy model and neurobehavioral approach.

Developmental framework

Many books and handouts on FAS recommend a developmental approach, based on developmental psychology, even though most do not specify it as such and provide little theoretical background. Optimal human development generally occurs in identifiable stages (e.g., Jean Piaget's theory of cognitive development, Erik Erikson's stages of psychosocial development, John Bowlby's attachment framework, and other developmental stage theories). FAS interferes with normal development, which may cause stages to be delayed, skipped, or immaturely developed. Over time, an unaffected child can negotiate the increasing demands of life by progressing through stages of development normally, but not so for a child with FAS

By knowing what developmental stages and tasks children follow, treatment and interventions for FAS can be tailored to helping a patient meet developmental tasks and demands successfully If a patient is delayed in the adaptive behavior domain, for instance, then interventions would be recommended to target specific delays through additional education and practice (e.g., practiced instruction on tying shoelaces), giving reminders, or making accommodations (e.g., using slip-on shoes) to support the desired functioning level. This approach is an advance over behavioral interventions, because it takes the patient's developmental context into account while developing interventions.

Advocacy model

The advocacy model takes the point of view that someone is needed to actively mediate between the environment and the person with FAS.[3] Advocacy activities are conducted by an advocate (for example, a family member, friend, or case manager) and fall into three basic categories. An advocate for FAS: (1) interprets FAS and the disabilities that arise from it and explains it to the environment in which the patient operates, (2) engenders change or accommodation on behalf of the patient, and (3) assists the patient in developing and reaching attainable goals.[3]

The advocacy model is often recommended, for example, when developing an Individualized Education Program (IEP) for the patient's progress at school.[50]

An understanding of the developmental framework would presumably inform and enhance the advocacy model, but advocacy also implies interventions at a systems level as well, such as educating schools, social workers, and so forth on best practices for FAS. However, several organizations devoted to FAS also use the advocacy model at a community practice level as well

Neurobehavioral approach

The neurobehavioral approach focuses on the neurological underpinnings from which behaviors and cognitive processes arise. It is an integrative perspective that acknowledges and encourages a multi-modal array of treatment interventions that draw from all FAS treatment approaches. The neurobehavioral approach is a serious attempt at shifting single-perspective treatment approaches into a new, coherent paradigm that addresses the complexities of problem behaviors and cognitions emanating from the CNS damage of FAS.

The neurobehavioral approach's main proponent is Diane Malbin, MSW, a recognized speaker and trainer in the FASD field, who first articulated the approach with respect to FASD and characterizes it as *"Trying differently rather than trying harder.* "The idea to *try differently* refers to trying different perspectives and intervention options based on effects of the CNS damage and particular needs of the patient, rather than *trying harder* at implementing behavioral-based interventions that have consistently failed over time to produce improved outcomes for a patient. This approach also encourages more strength-based interventions, which allow a patient to develop positive outcomes by promoting success linked to the patient's strengths and interests

Public health and policy

Treating FAS at the public health and public policy levels promotes FAS prevention and diversion of public resources to assist those with FAS.[3] It is related to the advocacy model but promoted at a systems level (rather than with the individual or family), such as developing community education and supports, state or province level prevention efforts (e.g., screening for maternal alcohol use during OB/GYN or prenatal medical care visits), or national awareness programs. Several organizations and state agencies in the U.S. are dedicated to this type of intervention

Prognosis

Primary disabilities

The primary disabilities of FAS are the functional difficulties with which the child is born as a result of CNS damage due to prenatal alcohol exposure. Often, primary disabilities are mistaken as *behavior problems*, but the underlying CNS damage is the originating source of a functional difficulty, rather than a mental health condition, which is considered a secondary disability.

The exact mechanisms for functional problems of primary disabilities are not always fully understood, but animal studies have begun to shed light on some correlates between functional problems and brain structures damaged by prenatal alcohol exposure. Representative examples include:

> ➤ Learning impairments are associated with impaired dendrites of the hippocampus

> ➤ Impaired motor development and functioning are associated with reduced size of the cerebellum

> ➤ Hyperactivity is associated with decreased size of the corpus callosum

Functional difficulties may result from CNS damage in more than one domain, but common functional difficulties by domain include. Note that this is not an exhaustive list of difficulties.

> ➤ Achievement — Learning disabilities

> ➤ Adaptive behavior — Poor impulse control, poor personal boundaries, poor anger management, stubbornness, intrusive behavior, too friendly with strangers, poor daily living skills, developmental delays

> ➤ Attention — Attention-Deficit/Hyperactivity Disorder (ADHD), poor attention or concentration, distractible

> ➤ Cognition — Intellectual disability, confusion under pressure, poor abstract skills, difficulty distinguishing between fantasy and reality, slower cognitive processing

> ➤ Executive functioning — Poor judgment, Information-processing disorder, poor at perceiving patterns, poor cause and effect reasoning, inconsistent at linking words to actions, poor generalization ability

> ➤ Language — Expressive or receptive language disorders, grasp parts but not whole concepts, lack understanding of metaphor, idioms, or sarcasm

> ➤ Memory — Poor short-term memory, inconsistent memory and knowledge base

> ➤ Motor skills — Poor handwriting, poor fine motor skills, poor gross motor skills, delayed motor skill development (e.g., riding a bicycle at appropriate age)

> ➤ Sensory processing and soft neurological problems — sensory processing disorder, sensory defensiveness, under sensitivity to stimulation

> ➤ Social communication — Intrude into conversations, inability to read nonverbal or social cues, "chatty" but without substance

Secondary disabilities

The secondary disabilities of FAS are those that arise later in life secondary to CNS damage. These disabilities often emerge over time due to a mismatch between the primary disabilities and environmental expectations; secondary disabilities can be ameliorated with early interventions and appropriate supportive services.[5]

Six main secondary disabilities were identified in a University of Washington research study of 473 subjects diagnosed with FAS, PFAS (partial fetal alcohol syndrome), and ARND (alcohol-related neurodevelopmental disorder):

> - Mental health problems — Diagnosed with ADHD, Clinical Depression, or other mental illness, experienced by over 90% of the subjects
> - Disrupted school experience — Suspended or expelled from school or dropped out of school, experienced by 60% of the subjects (age 12 and older)
> - Trouble with the law — Charged or convicted with a crime, experienced by 60% of the subjects (age 12 and older)
> - Confinement — For inpatient psychiatric care, inpatient chemical dependency care, or incarcerated for a crime, experienced by about 50% of the subjects (age 12 and older)
> - Inappropriate sexual behavior — Sexual advances, sexual touching, or promiscuity, experienced by about 50% of the subjects (age 12 and older)
> - Alcohol and drug problems — Abuse or dependency, experienced by 35% of the subjects (age 12 and older)

Two additional secondary disabilities exist for adult patients:

> - Dependent living — Group home, living with family or friends, or some sort of assisted living, experienced by 80% of the subjects (age 21 and older)
> - Problems with employment — Required ongoing job training or coaching, could not keep a job, unemployed, experienced by 80% of the subjects (age 21 and older)

Protective factors and strengths

Eight factors were identified in the same study as universal protective factors that reduced the incidence rate of the secondary disabilities.

> - Living in a stable and nurturing home for over 73% of life
> - Being diagnosed with FAS before age six
> - Never having experienced violence
> - Remaining in each living situation for at least 2.8 years

> ➢ Experiencing a "good quality home" (meeting 10 or more defined qualities) from age 8 to 12 years old

> ➢ Having been found eligible for developmental disability (DD) services

> ➢ Having basic needs met for at least 13% of life

> ➢ Having a diagnosis of FAS (rather than another FASD condition)

Malbin (2002) has identified the following areas of interests and talents as strengths that often stand out for those with FASD and should be utilized, like any strength, in treatment planning:

> ➢ Music, playing instruments, composing, singing, art, spelling, reading, computers, mechanics, woodworking, skilled vocations (welding, electrician, etc.), writing, poetry

> ➢ Participation in non-impact sport or physical fitness activities

History

Historical references

Anecdotal accounts of prohibitions against maternal alcohol use from Biblical, ancient Greek, and ancient Roman sources imply a historical awareness of links between maternal alcohol use and negative child outcomes.[35] In Gaelic Scotland, the mother and nurse were not allowed to consume ale during pregnancy and breastfeeding (Martin Martin).

The earliest recorded observation of possible links between maternal alcohol use and fetal damage was made in 1899 by Dr. William Sullivan, a Liverpool prison physician who noted higher rates of stillbirth for 120 alcoholic female prisoners than their sober female relatives; he suggested the causal agent to be alcohol use.[60] This contradicted the predominating belief at the time that heredity caused intellectual disability, poverty, and criminal behavior, which contemporary studies on the subjects usually concluded. A case study by Henry H. Goddard of the Kallikak family — popular in the early 1900s — represents this earlier perspective, though later researchers have suggested that the Kallikaks almost certainly had FAS. General studies and discussions on alcoholism throughout the mid-1900s were typically based on a heredity argument. Prior to fetal alcohol syndrome being specifically identified and named in 1973, a few studies had noted differences between the children of mothers who used alcohol during pregnancy or breast-feeding and those who did not, but identified alcohol use as a possible contributing factor rather than heredity.

Recognition as a syndrome

Fetal Alcohol Syndrome was named in 1973 by two dysmorphologists, Drs. Kenneth Lyons Jones and David Weyhe Smith of the University of Washington Medical School in Seattle, United States. They identified a pattern of "craniofacial, limb, and cardiovascular defects associated with prenatal onset growth deficiency and developmental delay" in eight unrelated children of three ethnic groups, all born to mothers who were alcoholics. The pattern of malformations indicated that the damage was prenatal. News of the discovery shocked some, while others were skeptical of the findings.[65]

Dr. Paul Lemoine of Nantes, France had already published a study in a French medical journal in 1968 about children with distinctive features whose mothers were alcoholics,[2]and in the U.S., Christy Ulleland and colleagues at the University of Washington Medical School[1] had conducted an 18-month study in 1968–1969 documenting the risk of maternal alcohol consumption among the offspring of 11 alcoholic mothers. The Washington and Nantes findings were confirmed by a research group in Gothenburg, Sweden in 1979.[66] Researchers in France, Sweden, and the United States were struck by how similar these children looked, though they were not related, and how they behaved in the same unfocused and hyperactive manner.

Within nine years of the Washington discovery, animal studies, including non-human monkey studies carried out at the University of Washington Primate Center by Dr. Sterling Clarren, had confirmed that alcohol was a teratogen. By 1978, 245 cases of FAS had been reported by medical researchers, and the syndrome began to be described as the most frequent known cause of intellectual disability.

While many syndromes are eponymous, i.e. named after the physician first reporting the association of symptoms, Dr. Smith named FAS after the causal agent of the symptoms.[67] He reasoned that doing so would encourage prevention, believing that if people knew maternal alcohol consumption caused the syndrome, then abstinence during pregnancy would follow from patient education and public awareness.[67] Nobody was aware of the full range of possible birth defects from FAS or its prevalence rate at that time, but admission of alcohol use during pregnancy can feel stigmatizing to birth mothers and complicate diagnostic efforts of a syndrome with its preventable cause in the name. Over time, as subsequent research and clinical experience suggested that a range of effects (including physical, behavioral, and cognitive) could arise from prenatal alcohol exposure, the term Fetal Alcohol Spectrum Disorder (FASD) was developed to include FAS as well as other conditions resulting from prenatal alcohol exposure. Currently, FAS is the only expression of prenatal alcohol exposure defined by the International Statistical Classification of Diseases and Related Health Problems and assigned ICD-9 and diagnoses.

BY HENRY AFRICA   **51**

CHAPTER 9 NINE

WHAT KIND OF FUTURE DO I FACE

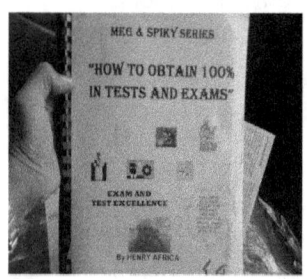

Just because you have been diagnosed with FETAL ALCOHOL SYNDROME does not mean you cannot rise above your circumstances… You require guts to achieve glory for yourself…
You can achieve whatever you set your mind to. Just remain focused and concentrate on what your goal in life is…CONCENTRATION is important…Many FAS sufferers get 100% grades.

This sweater says it all. It is possible to overcome anything that may hold you back. If you do not do it then it cannot be because you did not try…
We all have to overcome some challenge in life. If yours is difficult, don't think you have the worse set of challenges to overcome. Sometimes the grass is really greener on the other side…
GIVE IT YOUR ALL AND DON'T GIVE UP…

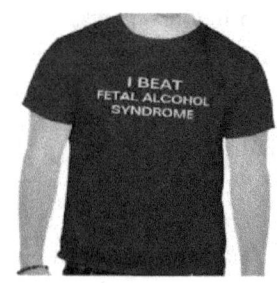

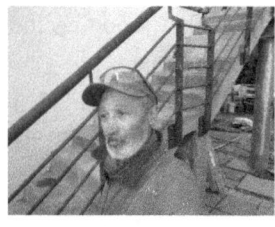

If you think that life is easier when you are born without FAS, then you may be a little bit mistaken. There are many other challenges that others have to face. You have a set of challenges but we ALL have some difficulty to overcome at some stage of our lives. There are many things that can go wrong during your life…

SUMMARY:

No one's future is a certainty. It is up to us to make the most of the hand we have been dealt with. If we simply surrender the hand then we will have no chance of coming out victorious. It takes effort and courage to face life with a start that is less than the best.
BUT THERE IS NO GUARANTEE THAT IF THINGS WERE BETTER TO START WITH, THAT IT WOULD MAKE THE END BETTER…

LIFE DOES NOT COME WITH GUARANTEES…

"THERE IS A TIDE IN THE AFFAIRS OF MAN WHICH TAKEN AT THE FLOOD LEADS ON TO FORTUNE; OMITTED ALL THEIR LIVES IS SPENT IN SHALLOWS AND IN MISERIES"

Oliver Wendell Homes

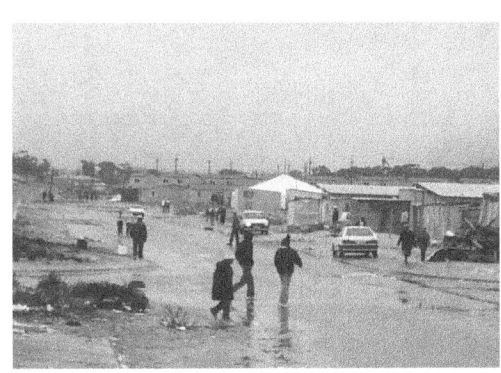 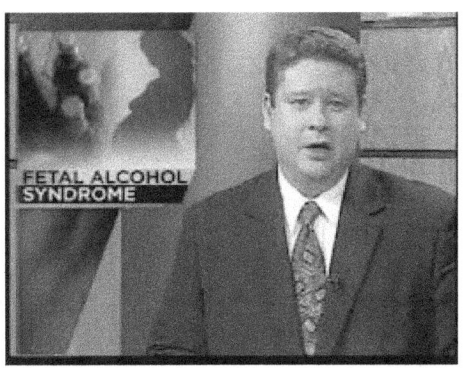

IT IS POSSIBLE FOR YOU TO OVERCOME ANY ADVERSE SET OF CIRCUMSTANCES. YOU WERE CREATED BY GOD TO BE VICTORIOUS...

It does not matter if you have challenges that appear to be a stumbling block to your future success. You have to overcome what you foresee in the immediate future. It is not going to be easy. You have to take control every day of your lives. It is no good blaming anyone else for the situation that you find yourself in.

FREEDOM FROM EMOTIONS allows us to succeed at life. Free the one who thinks they are to blame for where you are and you free yourself to move forward to achieve your success...

BY HENRY AFRICA   **53**

CHAPTER 9 NINE

WHAT KIND OF FUTURE DO I FACE

I BREAK WITH THE WAY THIS SERIES IS DONE TO INCLUDE A FEW PAGES FROM AN ARTICLE THAT I READ. CAN IT HELP YOU? I AM SURE THE WRITERS BELOW, WHO PENNED THE ARTICLE, WOULD AGREE TO PUBLISH IT AS WIDELY AS POSSIBLE TO BE ABLE TO HELP PEOPLE TO COPE... I have done minimal editing to this article...ALL CREDIT GOES TO THE PERSONS BELOW...

***** START *****

Fetal Alcohol Syndrome

Written by Teresa Bergen and Winnie Yu | Medically Reviewed by Jennifer Wider, MD

What Is Fetal Alcohol Syndrome?

*Women who drink alcohol during pregnancy can give birth to babies with **fetal alcohol spectrum disorders**. These disorders range from mild to severe. They can be behavioral, physical, related to learning, or all of the above.*

*Fetal **alcohol syndrome** (FAS) is a severe form of the condition. People with FAS may have problems with their vision, hearing, memory, attention span, and abilities to learn and communicate. While the defects vary from one person to another, the damage is often permanent.*

Causes of Fetal Alcohol Syndrome

When a pregnant woman drinks alcohol, some of that alcohol easily passes across the placenta to the fetus. The body of a developing fetus does not process alcohol the same way as an adult's. The alcohol is more concentrated in the fetus, and can prevent enough nutrition and oxygen from getting to the fetus' vital organs.

Damage can be done in the first few weeks of pregnancy when a woman might not yet know that she is pregnant. The risk increases if the mother is a heavy drinker.

According to many studies, alcohol use appears to be most harmful during the first three months of pregnancy. However, <u>consumption of alcohol</u> during any time during pregnancy can be harmful.

Symptoms of Fetal Alcohol Syndrome

Since fetal alcohol <u>syndrome</u> covers a wide range of problems, there are many possible <u>symptoms</u>. The severity of these symptoms ranges from mild to severe, and can include:

- *a <u>small head</u>*
- *a smooth ridge between the <u>upper lip</u> and <u>nose</u>, small eyes, a very thin upper lip, or other abnormal <u>facial features</u>*
- *below-average height and weight*
- *hyperactivity*
- *lack of focus*
- *poor coordination*
- *<u>delayed development</u> and problems in thinking, speech, movement and <u>social skills</u>*
- *poor judgment*
- *problems seeing or hearing*
- *learning disabilities*
- *mental retardation*
- *heart problems*
- *<u>kidney</u> defects and abnormalities*
- *deformed limbs or fingers*
- *mood swings*

Diagnosing Fetal Alcohol Syndrome

Early <u>diagnosis</u> can increase a positive outcome in the child. Talk to your doctor if you think your child might have FAS. Let your doctor know if you drank while you were pregnant.

A <u>physical exam</u> of the baby may show a <u>heart murmur</u> or other <u>heart problems</u>. As the baby matures, there may be other signs that help confirm the diagnosis, these include:

- *slow rate of growth*
- *abnormal facial features or bone growth*
- *hearing and <u>vision problems</u>*
- *slow <u>language acquisition</u>*

BY HENRY AFRICA   **55**

> small *head size*
> poor coordination

To diagnose an individual with FAS, the doctor must determine that he or she has abnormal facial features, slower than normal growth, and central nervous system problems. These nervous system problems could be physical or behavioral. They might present as hyperactivity, lack of coordination or focus or learning disabilities.

Treating Fetal Alcohol Syndrome

While FAS is incurable, some symptoms can be treated. The earlier the diagnosis, the more progress is likely to be made.

Special education and social services can help very young children. For example, speech therapists can work with toddlers to help them learn to talk. Children with FAS will benefit from a stable and loving home. FAS children can be even more sensitive to disruptions in routine than an average child. FAS children are especially likely to develop problems with violence and substance abuse later in life if they are exposed to violence or abuse at home. These children do well with a regular routine, simple rules to follow, and rewards for positive behavior.

Depending on what type of symptoms the FAS child exhibits, he or she may need many doctor or specialist visits. There are no medications that specifically treat FAS. However, several medications may address symptoms.

These medications include:

> **antidepressants** to treat problems with sadness and negativity
> **stimulants** to treat lack of focus, hyperactivity, and other behavioral problems
> **neuroleptics** to treat anxiety and aggression
> **anti-anxiety drugs** to treat anxiety

Behavioral training may also help FAS children. For instance, friendship training teaches kids social skills for interacting with their peers. Executive function training may improve skills such as self-control, reasoning, and understanding cause and effect. Children with FAS might also need academic help. For example, a math tutor could help a child who struggles in school.

Parents and siblings might also need help in dealing with the challenges this condition can cause. This help can come through talk therapy or support groups. Parents can also receive parental training tailored to the needs of those with FAS children. Parental training teaches you how to best interact with and care for your FAS child.

Some parents and their FAS children seek alternative treatments outside the medical establishment. These include healing practices, such as massage and acupuncture (the placement of thin needles into key body areas). Alternative treatments also include movement techniques, such as exercise or yoga.

Preventing Fetal Alcohol Syndrome

Fetal alcohol syndrome does not occur if the mother refrains from drinking during pregnancy. If you are a woman with a drinking problem who wants to get pregnant, seek help from a health care professional. If you are a light or social drinker, do not drink if you think you might become pregnant anytime soon. Remember, the effects of alcohol can make a mark during the first few weeks of a pregnancy.

***** END *****

SUMMARY:

As an interested person, I have to be honest about this book. I have had a warped understanding of what FAS is all about. Thanks to articles which I have read on the internet, I have been brought to a deeper understanding about what the disorder is all about. There can be no doubt that if my wife had fallen pregnant I would have been of the opinion in the past that it was ok for her to have a glass or two of wine during the 9 months of her pregnancy. My opinion about that has changed after all the research I have read. This book alone has made me understand the need to REFRAIN completely from drugs and substances of any kind during your pregnancy.

I took a girl in at one stage of my life. I had a big empty company home. It was there I first encountered the term heroine baby... My very young girlfriend had been a drug addict who would do whatever it took to stay on the road and hid the fact that she was doing HEROINE or UNGA as it was called in South Africa. No amount of counselling helped her to give up the habit. There were times she just disappeared and then would re-appear as if nothing was out of the ordinary. Julie would not even realize how much time had passed since she had left home. A week was the same like a day to her.

I could not live with her and sent her back to her family very soon after she started doing drugs in our home. I had one strict rule and she broke it... NO DRUGS AT HOME...

CHAPTER 10 TEN

WILL I HATE YOU TOMORROW MOTHER?

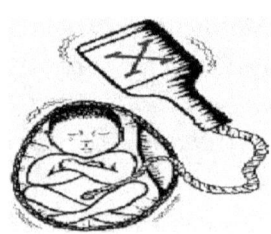

"Didn't you know that there was the possibility that I would be born deformed if you drank during your pregnancy Mom? I am told that the chance of a brain damaged child is high when you have been drinking excessively during your pregnancy. Why didn't you try and stop Mom... Didn't you love me enough to make the effort?

"My child could hate me if he or she is born deformed. I have no control over how I feel towards the unborn baby. Her father forced me to have sex one night and he knew I didn't want to have children so he forced himself on me when he knew I wasn't taking birth control. I am going to drink until I lose this child... A natural abortion...

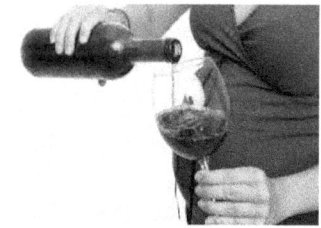

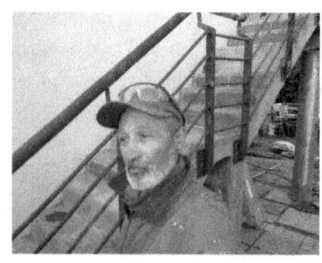

I would be the last person to judge your behavior. Your reason for doing what you are doing is good enough and makes sense. But have you thought about some other alternatives. How about separation and then giving the child up for adoption? You can also divorce and then place a healthy born child up for adoption...The child does not have to suffer does it? For their whole life if they make it to be born with FAS...

SUMMARY:

I am not going to have all the answers but I think every person needs to find the solution that best deals with their own set of circumstances. Don't make hasty and emotional decisions and join a support group that can help you cope with the set of circumstances you are facing. Hasty decisions have the habit of coming back to haunt you for a long time. No one can stop you from taking whatever course you choose. It is your body and what happens in that body is your responsibility as a woman. Men cannot dictate to you what and how you do things relating to your body...

HAVING CHILDREN IS A RESPONSIBILITY THAT GOD WILL REQUIRE AN ACOUNT OF.
No one else can dictate to you what you should do...JUST GET ADVICE OK...

"IT'S EASY TO MAKE FUN OF A SITUATION UNTIL YOU ARE ON THE RECEIVING END. THEN THE FUN FLIES OUT OF THE WINDOW AND THE TRAGEDY FLIES IN"

By ANONYOMUS

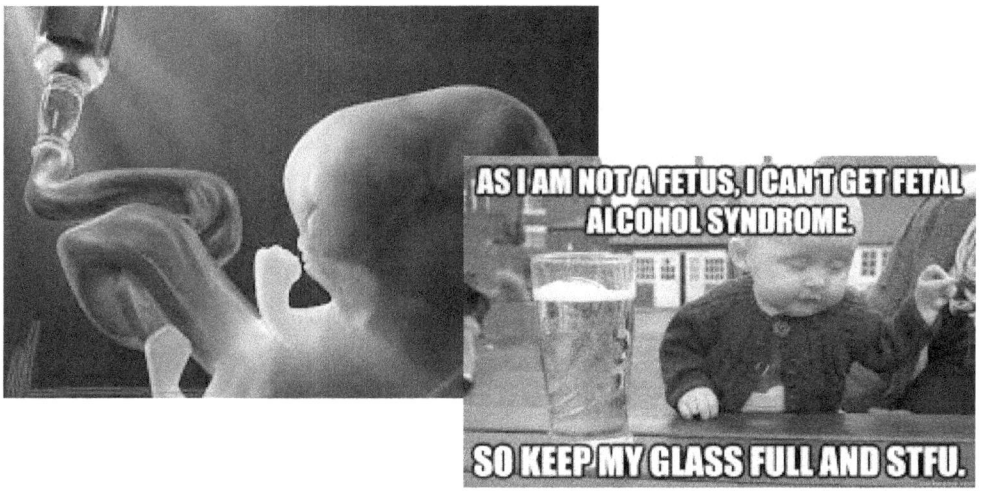

Keep that glass full long enough during the time you are pregnant and it is almost a foregone conclusion that the child with the witty comment is going to look a little different. He may look a little like the pictures that are spread all over these pages.

You may love them just a little less because they will be a constant reminder of your inability to take life SERIOUSLY… FETAL ALCOHOL SYNDROME IS A REALITY…

DON'T PLAY RUSSIAN ROULETTE WITH THE FUTURE OF YOUR UNBORN CHILD…

CHAPTER 10 TEN

WILL I HATE YOU TOMORROW MOTHER

I found out over the last few months that my mother also drank during her pregnancy. She did it in moderation and did not get stoned like some pregnant mothers who drown their babies in alcohol every day. Now what is moderation? They have almost concluded that 1 to 2 glasses of standard glasses of wine will not damage the unborn child's brain cells or restrict their growth in any way. Now there are studies and there are studies. Will one in the future find that a select group of children, who are only exposed to 1 glass of wine a day, end up with brain damaged assigned to the pre-natal stage? I think if you can drop your alcohol level to 1 or 2 glasses then you may as well quit the habit for 9 months or quit getting knocked up. I read about this woman who lives in a wendy house/fema trailer who has 12 children with 8 of them still living with her. Man is that going overboard or what? Somehow there needs to be some laws like in China about having 1 child. Ok so maybe 2 or 3 in South Africa is practical. But 12 children? My grand-mother had 11...But then they never had television at that stage in 1929...I am sure many children who have a basic mental capacity will grow to hate their parents in one way or another. Maybe even in patches if not completely. It's inevitable if they find you are responsible for turning them into a circus freak by your undisciplined drinking while you were pregnant that they would hold it against you... Wouldn't you expect that to be the case? You would have deprived them of an ordinary life and an ordinary family existence, free of doctors and medical bills, free of pointing fingers and laughs behind their backs... Free of hurtful comments and abuse for being different...

SUMMARY

Cannot say this will definitely happen if they are diagnosed with FAS, but what do you really think should be the treatment you receive if you have been irresponsible during your pregnancy. It is after all only 9 months. You can do it. You can abstain. You fight every addiction with God's help. It is worth the struggle if you really want to be guaranteed of having a normal child when you give birth. If you partied until you found out you were pregnant, b accident, then you have already drowned your child in alcohol through the pre=natal phase. That should be enough to get you concerned about what kind of fetus will be growing in your womb. I am going to answer a question posed to me honestly. Would I hate my mother if she drank and I was born deformed? YES!!! Without a shadow of a doubt would be my answer. The selfishness of her act would be something I would not be able to forgive if I actually had any brain ability. You see, you actually need brain ability to hate. Without a brain, there is no capacity to hate. Maybe in that way a child with an IQ of less than 25 will be better than a child who has an IQ of over 25... There is a huge difference in their abilities given an IQ point or two...

AND IT ALLCOMES DOWN TO A DECISION YOU CAN MAKE AHEAD OF TIME...

CHAPTER 11 ELEVEN

FREAK IN A CIRCUS SHOW-KIDS FRIENDS VISIT

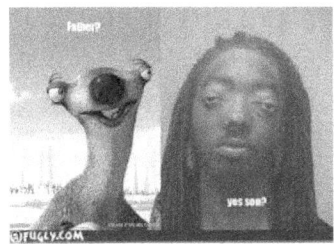

I am not sure how this picture originated but the comparison may offend some people. I think Sid did become a hero of sorts in the ICE AGE movie series.

We will find the most unlikely people become heroes during our lives.

YOU BECOME A HERO FOR OTHERS

Any child can end up having Fetal Alcohol Syndrome. The disorder comes about because of the abuse of alcohol during the pregnancy of your mother. You have no say in her behavior while you are inside her womb....

If a pregnant woman drinks alcohol, she is putting her unborn baby at risk. Would you?

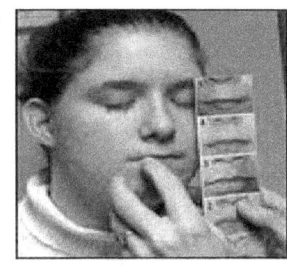

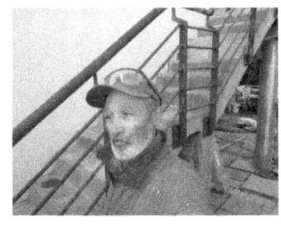

Kids will say the darndest things. They are going to say things that will hurt you deeply. Most of the time they are just trying to make sense of what they see for the first time.

"Why do you look so funny and your parents are normal?" said with no malicious intent is going to cut you to the heart... DON'T TAKE IT PERSONALLY... THE TRUTH SETS YOU

SUMMARY:

It was not your fault was it? Did you do the drinking or did your mother? Now you think you can live your life justifying her mistake for her. The answer to the statement is simple... "I HAVE FAS CAUSED BY MY MOTHER DRINKING DURING HER PREGNANCY" And you will have to live with hearing that every time you do... The reality is that you DID drink and you knew better. You were warned by so many people during the 9 months that you were pregnant. There is no guilt due to your child. And why should she defend you? You didn't want to listen...

LEARN TO ACCEPT YOUR MISTAKE. IT WILL MAKE LIFE EASIER FOR EVERYONE... THEY WILL LEARN A LESSON TOO...

"I SAW THE FUTURE BUT I COULDN'T EMBRACE IT BECAUSE I WAS TRAPPED IN THE PAST"

Henri Michael

Diagnosis (1973)

- Prenatal and Postnatal growth retardation
- Neurological Abnormalities
  - developmental delays
  - behavioral dysfunction
  - intellectual impairment
  - skull or brain malformations
- Characteristic Facial Features
  - Skin folds at eye corner
  - Small head circumference
  - Small eye opening
  - Thin upper lip
  - Indistinct philtrum

It will come down to how hard you try for 1 year. From the time you find out you want a child and then become pregnant, you WILL have to make the choice to be responsible. There is no other way to give your child the best chance to be born healthy…

LIFE IS MADE UP OF CHOICES… NO ONE CAN MAKE THIS ONE FOR YOU… YOU MUST WANT A DIFFERENT FUTURE…

BY HENRY AFRICA   **62**

CHAPTER 11 ELEVEN

FREAK IN A CIRCUS SHOW-KIDS FRIENDS VISIT

Getting the role of Sid in the movie ICE AGE could be something special if you had an IQ of 25 or in that region. Getting it if you have an IQ of around 150 could be an insult to some. Now if I was say, Charlie Sheen then I could do a role like that. Purely based on my behavior in the past. Having behaved so badly that people may think he had FAS as a child. But did he have it or not... maybe he did. But will that make a difference in his ability to become wealthy? No it did not do that for him. He ended up winning and that means that so can you. You do not have to let the circumstances that affected many millions of others, condemn you to a life as a vegetable in a cabbage patch. There is intelligence in every human being. It may surprise us in the future when we come to understand the many levels people can communicate on.

Until we came to understand right and left brain ability, Einstein was called a stupid child... Vincent van Gogh was called mentally retarded [Challenged today]. The list goes on...And on and on...

SUMMARY

This world favors right brained analytical people like me. But there are so many amazing people who have left brain abilities. They are the artistic creative geniuses we have to patiently teach to do different thing. Without patience they will not be able to achieve what they can in life. One lost Michelangelo or Leonardo da Vinci can rob us of a talent that could have made out world a better place to live in. The inventors who discovered electricity, radiology and many other important things were thought to be crazy.

If that is the case then I would rather be grouped with the crazy bunch of people because the way I see it there was much more talent in that group than the rest of the world of right brain thinkers. We call them movers and shakers. But how much talent does it take to be an artist. If you have that talent then your painting will sell for millions... Unfortunately it will only happen after you are long dead... That's the sad part of that scenario.

Connect on the golfing course and you can make the stash today. Tennis can pretty much get you an early retirement. And don't tell me that because of FAS you cannot do it. I am starting to believe that anything you put your mind to you can do...

THAT ABILITY TO ACTUALIZE IS NOT RESTRICTED TO WHOM WE CALL NORMAL PEOPLE. GOD IS THERE TO MAKE EVERYONE ANYTHING THEY WANT TO... GO OUT AND MAKE THE BEST OF YOUR LIFE ON EARTH...
YOU WERE DESIGNED BY A GOD THAT CREATED YOU TO BE A WINNER...

CHAPTER 12 TWELVE
MY PERFECT SPOUSE NOT MINE ANYMORE

VIEW 1

It is easy for other people to judge without understanding what is involved in the process that leads a mother to continue drinking alcohol while she is pregnant. There are reasons why she **DOES NOT** quit the drinking. Dealing with those reasons means helping to resolve the problem.

DON'T JUDGE TOO QUICKLY...

FACT

Fetal alcohol syndrome is a disorder that is the result of abuse of alcohol during pregnancy. It is 100% preventable. A pregnant woman plays Russian roulette when she ingests alcohol ...

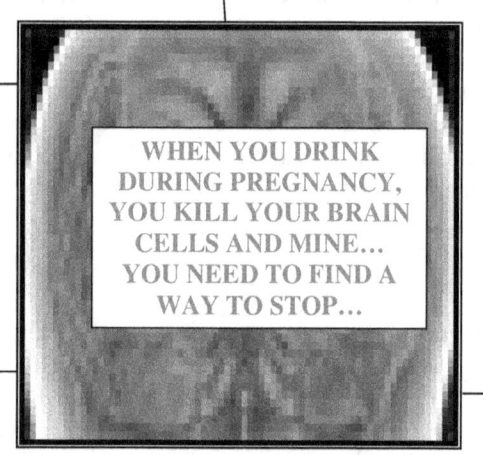

WHEN YOU DRINK DURING PREGNANCY, YOU KILL YOUR BRAIN CELLS AND MINE... YOU NEED TO FIND A WAY TO STOP...

FACT

PEOPLE WHO HOLD GRUDGES BURN THEMSELVES OUT BY ALWAYS NEEDING FUEL TO KEEP THAT FIRE BURNING. IT IS BETTER TO LET GO AND MOVE ON... THAT'S THE WAY GOD WANTS US TO LIVE...MOVE ON I SAY...

VIEW 2

My mother's selfish behavior has physically deformed me. She knew the risks when she refused to listen to friends who warned her about drinking while she was pregnant with me. H could she do that? My whole future is going to be different because of her behavior.

Who will want to go out with me the way I look now. It need not have been this way...

THIS REGRET COULD DRIVE YOU INSANE. YOU MUST FORGIVE

SUMMARY:

It's a hard process to change habits that you become used to. There is a thought process connected to every action we perform. Triggers are set in place and after an event then the trigger is activated and the body instructs the brain how to feel. We cannot give in to those feelings if we are going to conquer addictions. Yes, its addiction that is the danger. Regular and continual use of harmful substances leads to addiction. Our body then needs the chemicals we ingest on a regular basis.

WE NEED TO FIND A WAY TO OVERCOME THAT DEPENDANCY. IT IS CRITICAL WE DO...

BY HENRY AFRICA

"LIFE BRINGS YOU TO MANY CROSSROADS. REST AT THAT CROSSROADS BUT DON'T YOU QUIT. THE CROWN OF VICTORY GOES TO THE ONE WHO PERSEVERES"

By Henry Africa

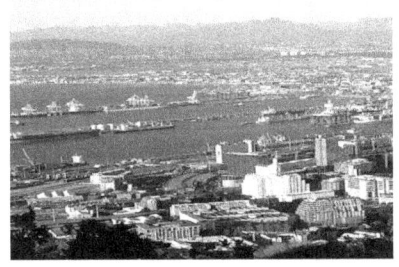

CAPE TOWN SOUTH AFRICA

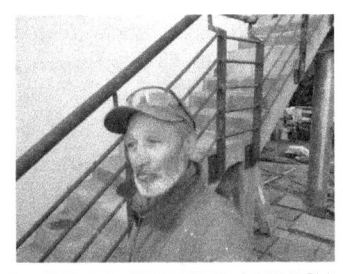

AUTHOR HENRY AFRICA

IS THIS A TAG YOU WOULD LIKE TO HAVE BELOW YOUR NAME? THE ONE CAPE TOWN IS WHAT I AM REFERRING TO ACTUALLY. I AM HAPPY WITH MY TAG… I EARNED THAT TAG DIDN'T I? BUT WHAT WERE THE TAGS I HAD BEFORE THE ONES LIKE AUTHOR WERE PLACED THERE?

- LEGENDARY BASEBALL PLAYER
- SMART BUSINESS MAN
- PROPERTY DEVELOPER
- SEDAN TAXI DRIVER…
- PUBLISHING COMPANY OWNER…

"I AM A WORK IN PROGRESS LIKE EACH OF YOU. IF YOU HAVE FAS THEN YOU STILL HAVE WORK TO DO TO ESTABLISH YOUR CREDENTIALS TOO. AN FAS DIAGNOSED BASEBALL PLAYER HIT A HOME RUN IN THE PRO LEAGUE IN THE USA. HE MADE IT I WOULD SAY… I NEVER DID… SO THAT TELLS ME THAT ALL IS NOT LOST FOR FAS SUFFERERS. THEY CAN ATTAIN ANY HEIGHT THEY WANT. THEY CAN DO EVEN BETTER THAN THOSE WHO THINK THEY ARE SO COOL AND ARE PART OF THE IN CROWD… EBERYONE DESERVES A CHANCE TO BECOME THE BEST…"

CHAPTER 12 TWELVE

MY PERFECT SPOUSE NOT MINE ANYMORE

Oh lets go on a date… You sound like such an amazing man. Maybe we are meant to be soul mates John. How about we go for coffee over the weekend. I believe you will be back here for the weekend from your holidays out in Sweden.

Ok, let's do that. I do have some time to spare between book signing engagements. Let's make it 8 o'clock on Friday evening at the Mug & Bean coffee shop in the waterfront. Will that be ok with you? Where shall I pick you up Kathryn…?

Its fine John. I will meet you at the coffee shop. Whoever gets there first can take a table and then will let the manager know where I am sitting or you let them know where you are sitting if you get there first. In any event one of us should check with the manager when we get there ok?

Ok with me Kathryn, Look forward to it…

It's a few days later now and Kohn has been on his date with Kathryn. Kathryn is a hot, blonde bombshell. John is the normal looking FAS sufferer you have seen. But he is different. So much so that it is obvious to anyone who knows that he looks different from most men. Kathryn never knew this and she was uncomfortable and immediately decided to end the date as quick as she could. Peer pressure meant she would not want to have a husband with FASD. She did not want to be stared at everywhere she went. Is Kathryn vain? What do you think?

SUMMARY

My heart breaks for John. He had hoped that he met the most awesome girl. Judging from her pictures he had seen. She assumed that John was a normal bloke and that he was as interesting as they came. He is very interesting and speaks so well. He is an amazing man with the most jovial nature. He would make the most amazing candidate for a great parent or father. But his eyes are spaced far apart and he is the typical FAS pictures you would see on a billboard. Society has come to judge this kind of person as being inferior to the "Normal" looking male jock.

Maybe Kathryn will rather end up married to a man who abuses her or cheats on her. But she is determined not to be stared at by everyone when she walks by her neighbors in the local mall. Is it possible that John can find a woman that has the same intellect level as he does without her judging him because of his looks?

It's very sad that we live in a society that bases its values on looks when God says we have to look at the heart. Can we become that way? Can we look at others and find out what kind of hearts they have. John's heart is so sooo open to love and to love deeply. Was Kathryn the wrong one for him? Maybe they should have got to know each other better before going on a date. Maybe then she may have looked deeper before throwing in the towel on their relationship. She could have been mine, if I didn't have Fetal Alcohol Syndrome… If I wasn't different from other men. Why God why did you make me….

EPILOGUE
REASONS OR EXCUSES

"THIS IS TAKEN FROM ONLINE WORK PUBLISHED BY SOMEONE ELSE. I TAKE NO CREDIT FOR THIS WORK... THIS CHAPTER IS CUT AND PASTED FOR THE GOOD OF MANY. If anyone has any issues with that then I will remove it before I launch Edition 1 proper"... Author Henry Africa

START

Continuing a partying lifestyle during pregnancy can have devastating and lifelong effects on children affected by their mothers' drinking and drugging. Heavy alcohol and drug use during pregnancy can cause birth defects for which there is no cure or treatment.

A visitor to our Alcoholism / Substance Abuse Forum described the long-term effects that his wife's heavy alcohol consumption and cocaine use throughout her pregnancy has had on their now 19-year-old son. Dave describes the guilt he now feels because of the struggles that his son may face for the rest of his life. All credit for the following story goes to Dave-Hope it helps you...

CAN THE FOLLOWING STORY CHANGE YOUR LIFE. IT HAS CHANGED MINE... ALL CREDIT GOES TO SOMEONE CALLED DAVE...

Dave's Story

I'm in my mid-40s now, and I've been clean and sober for almost 13 years. It's been a good recovery -- I was ready for sobriety, and haven't had any relapses or anything like that. Back when I was a kid I dropped out of college after five years and no degree, mostly because of a major marijuana problem. Heavy wine drinking came later. I moved two times zones away to get away from my family and friends (you don't want to be nagged about throwing your life away all the time, you know?) and just pretty much sat around getting stoned and drunk all the time.

Before long I met a nice girl with pretty much the same background and habits, and we got along just fine and began dating. One difference, though -- her drug of choice was cocaine, while I stayed true to marijuana. She drank rum, while I preferred cheap wine. We never fought, not once, and just enjoyed ourselves by working low-stress, easy jobs and hung out with our roommates and all just drank, smoked, snorted, drank, smoked, snorted, and all was well.

She Kept the Pregnancy Secret

Until nine months later when my girlfriend surprised me and everyone else we knew by giving birth to a (seemingly) healthy eight-pound boy. I admit I was very, very naive. Also, there were times I suspected that not all was right in my little world, and asked, obliquely, about "that-time-of-the-month" but was always assured everything was OK. Also, I was smoking about an ounce of weed a week, and drinking maybe a liter and a half of wine a night -- I was doing a pretty thorough job of drifting into oblivion. And oblivious I was. So life as it was just went on. Until my girlfriend drove herself to the hospital one day and had a baby.

Drinking, Smoking and Snorting

After 14 years, the marriage finally broke up. There are probably a dozen reasons the marriage failed, and it doesn't matter now, anyway.But one big problem we kept fighting over during those years was the first pregnancy. "Why didn't you tell me? How could you drink, smoke cigarettes, and snort cocaine knowing you were pregnant?" Her responses to those questions were rarely calm or satisfactory.

Son Kept Having Behavioral Problems

The issue kept coming up, however, because it did bother me that she kept the pregnancy a secret (even her friends were shocked) but also because our son kept having behavioral problems. We took him to counselors, read books, talked to people. Through it all my wife insisted that any trouble our son was having had nothing to do with any prenatal exposure to anything. When I insisted that we disclose the history to our pediatrician, it turned into an ugly argument, to say the least. No doctor or counselor suspected anything about the pregnancy as the culprit, which solidified my wife's conviction that there was no prenatal damage with our son. Depression runs in both families, kids will be kids, etc.

Nothing Is Working

He did well academically, too. His teachers liked him. He never got into trouble at school. He graduated high school just this past June, with a 3.79 grade point average. But all through the years he struggled with making friends and kept mostly to himself. He would cry a lot, and complain about being depressed. He's been on several antidepressants over the years. He's been in counseling for years. Nothing has worked. Our son made it through high school with fabulous grades. But at 19, he has few friends, still complains about depression, has taken to cutting himself and is prone to fits of anxiety and rage. He can't decide about college or not, and refuses to get a job no matter what we do. He goes to counseling. We have family sessions. We talk about college. We talk about getting a job. Nothing is making a difference.

Fetal Alcohol Syndrome

He can go from whistling a tune to smashing his laptop without warning. He has beaten the crap out of the dashboard of his car. He tears books apart, breaks appliances, snaps pencils, cuts himself, rips clothes. **He can also be kind and caring, peaceful and funny, remorseful and helpful. He's a good kid, with a soft heart.** I have always suspected fetal alcohol syndrome (he does not have the classic facial deformities of FAS) or some sort of brain damage from the cocaine. I no longer have any doubt. I've spent a lot of time this week reading about fetal alcohol syndrome and fetal alcohol spectrum disorder and other related syndromes. *He Will Never Have a Normal Life...* I mean, when you consider his gestational history, it is astonishing he was born alive and has done as well as he has. I am afraid this is not a phase; this is not a matter of changing medications, or giving him some uplifting literature. I am afraid he will never have a normal life. **He is paying the price for something he had no control over.** Something that never should have happened. Oh my God. I don't know how to help him. God, I am so sorry. I am so sorry.

-- Dave

END*

AUTHOR FOOTNOTE
ONLY A HABIT CAN SUPPRESS ANOTHER HABIT

I have a habit. I love to sleep around with women. Anyone who is on the make can get me into the sack. I have a problem. Must be addicted to sex. Is that a crime in the society I live in? Not really, unless you are a pastor and you have a church that looks up to you. It started by accident and quickly escalated into a habit that was out of control. I can now do 3 or 4 different women every night when I am out on the road. It's easy to find them. We live in a society where women will do anything to find a man with some ability to give them the things in life they want. We may call them many names but generally prostitute is a word that may best help to describe them.

But what about me? What am I as a man when I sleep around with women? Don't they have a name for me too? Why haven't I got a tag? Why has the woman got a tag that demeans her? She is doing this for a number of reasons. One is that she has no job and has a mother and a child to feed and house. Why then don't I help her because she has a valid reason to get help from me? I cannot afford to help her because I am not financially able to help every girl with a financial problem that goes to the street for help. I did try that for a while but then I got into sleeping with them and that led to me shacking up with one of them…. Then another one and another. It was a habit that quickly got out of hand…

I DEFINITEELY NEEDED A NEW HABIT. I KNOW THAT ONLY A HABIT CAN SUPPRESS ANOTHER HABIT…

What I describe above is a situation that John got into because he has got no luck to find the beautiful woman he so much desires. He has every skill that makes him a catch for the beautiful women of this world. But he is cursed to have FAS-Fetal Alcohol Syndrome and in our society is classed as a freak. There is no looking at the heart where this is concerned. Society looks down on anyone who is not perfect… Perfect on the outside anyway.
"I wish I were dead," John thinks to himself… "Why did you allow me to be made like this God?" he thinks as he drives along the main road. He stops when he sees Sandra standing on the side of the road…
"Sandra, want to go for a drive with me honey?" he says non chalantly

"Usual rates John," she says before getting into the beautiful Mercedes Benz.
"Sure Sandra...Money is no problem right, but you know that hey," he adds as an afterthought. Guess this is my destiny he thinks to himself. No decent girl will want to go out with me and get married to me... John has long given up on finding his pretty woman. He now resigns himself to being seen as a freak of nature because of the disorder he suffers from.

Sandra really can't understand why John thinks so little of himself. She thinks he is such an amazing man... So tender when he is with her and he never gets angry at anything she says or does. Sometimes she is impatient and then he simply shrugs and gets her something he remembers she always wanted. He does have lots of money but does not have any friends. Must be because he trusts people so little. Having been hurt by people's unkind remarks has that effect on anyone. They start to think that all people are just out to get something from you and then they show their true colors when any confrontation occurs and they make nasty statements that hurt to the core... The words FREAK and CIRCUS PERFORMER tend to be amongst those thrown around at that time... Extremely hurtful at times but more so when you are a person who has FAS. It's something like a dagger blow to your heart and soul. It is as if someone is twisting a knife blade inside of you. All you try to do is be a normal human being and it seems everyone is determined to make you feel lower than an animal in this world.

"Sandra how do you feel about going out with a guy like me some time," John says after careful thought. Sandra seems like she is different from the rest of the girls he has come to know. She is sensitive when she is with him. Perhaps she may even get to like him if she gets to know him, he thinks.
"What makes you think I would want to be seen in public with you John?" she purposely says.
"Everyone would stare at you and then you would get flustered and maybe fight with them, she adds... "Would you fight with them when you are out with me John? she asks seriously.
"Why would I do that Sandra? Johns asks innocently. At the best of times John really does not understand why society has to target him because of his different looks...
"Will you ask me to marry you John," Sandra asks seriously...Looking him straight in the eye.

BY HENRY AFRICA   **72**

"You are being funny with me right Sandra? John looks inquiringly at her.

No, I am being dead serious John," Sandra replies… "I have known you for a while now and I think perhaps we could make each other happy. The world does not subscribe to me and I have seen that you have a great heart and a kindness that comes from deep inside of you"

"Besides you stay alone in that big house and come to me every day so it will save you money if we move in and still do what we do every night…

"Why Sandra... Why would you marry a freak like me? The world will make you unhappy when you are with me. Society does not accept us FAS people. They see us as aliens amongst them."

"I guess I am different John," Sandra says with tears starting to appear in her eyes. She feels the pain that John must be feeling now… Years and years of rejection has eaten into his soul and poisoned what started out as a beautiful and pure soul….

It is 5 years later and John and Sandra celebrate their 5th Anniversary. Henry is there as he has been friends with Sandra and John for many years. He does not judge people and lives to help people everywhere, no matter how they look. He is the best friend you could have… He is prepared to die for his friends. If the situation has to arise… And Kathryn, his friend at the anniversary feels the same about her friends. Maybe they will be friends for the rest of their lives. They have been since the first time they met…

"Happy Anniversary John and Sandra," says Kathryn… Ole grumpy Henry dragged me with him on another wedding date. Seems to be a habit of his. Wonder if he is trying to give me some kind of message or something, "she says laughing. Kathryn laughs so easily, thinks Henry. She would make any guy a great wife… Maybe soon Kathryn will find the man she can be happy with…

"Can you bring the goodies in Henry? I packed a bag of things for John and Sandra... It's in the trunk. Be a luv and get them for us."

"Anything for you Kathryn," says Henry…And bring the ring in the glove campartment too Henry. I have decided to ask you to marry me tonight. I can't wait on you anymore. If I keep on waiting then I am going to be old and grey before you ask me… I think its time Henry... We are not getting any younger…"Yes Kathryn," says Henry nonchalantly… "Kathryn will always get what Kathryn wants," he thinks too himself and smiles as he goes to the car…   THE END

BY HENRY AFRICA   **73**

WARNING
MEDICAL PEOPLE DID NOT CAUSE THE DISORDER, THEY ARE JUST TRYING TO HELP

Antioxidants May Help Prevent Birth Defects Tied to Alcohol

Can Diminish the Incidence of Major Malformations

By UNC School of Medicine

Updated June 19, 2004

"THIS IS TAKEN FROM ONLINE WORK PUBLISHED BY SOMEONE ELSE. I TAKE NO CREDIT FOR THIS WORK… THIS CHAPTER IS CUT AND PASTED FOR THE GOOD OF MANY. If anyone has any issues with that then I will remove it before I launch Edition 1 proper"… Author Henry Africa

START Pregnant women who abuse alcohol may reduce the risk of birth defects in their babies by taking antioxidants during pregnancy, a University of North Carolina at Chapel Hill study indicates.

The new research found a 36 percent reduction in limb malformations in the offspring of pregnant mice exposed to ethanol and at the same time given a newly developed antioxidant compound called EUK-134.

The study appears on-linein FASEB-J, the journal of the Federation of American Societies for Experimental Biology. "What makes this study unique is that it shows for the first time that giving antioxidants to a pregnant mother at the same time she's exposed to alcohol can diminish the incidence of major malformations," said Dr. Kathleen K. Sulik, professor of cell and developmental biology at UNC's School of Medicine. Antioxidants protect key cellular components by neutralizing the damaging effects of free radicals, natural byproducts of cell metabolism. Free radicals form when oxygen is metabolized, or burned off, by the body. They travel through cells, disrupting the structure of other molecules, causing cellular damage. Such cell damage is believed to contribute to aging and various health problems. Examples of antioxidants are selenium, vitamin C and E, zinc and superoxide dismutase (or SOD), a zinc- and copper- or manganese-containing enzyme that reacts with superoxide radicals to convert them to less dangerous chemical entities.

Alcohol Kills Embryonic Cells

Dietary antioxidants have attracted considerable interest in the popular press as potential treatments for cancer, atherosclerosis, chronic inflammatory disease and aging. Sulik, a member of the university's Bowles Center for Alcohol Studies, said a major focus of her research has been cellular mechanisms involved in birth defect formation, particularly those linked to ethanol exposure, such as fetal alcohol spectrum disorders, or FASD. Until now, much of this research at UNC and elsewhere has involved growing cells in the laboratory. "We have used embryonic neural crest cells, which are very sensitive to ethanol," said Dr. Shao-yu Chen, a member of the Bowles Center for Alcohol Studies, assistant professor of cell and developmental biology and lead author of the new report.

"In a cell culture system, ethanol induces the death of these cells. But when we place antioxidants into the culture together with ethanol, the cells are protected from cell death." Chen also has shown that ethanol-induced cell death is related to free radical generation. "We have used superoxide dismutase and vitamin E and found that in the presence of ethanol both agents reduce free radical production," he said. Chen and Sulik have extended their cell culture research to a whole embryo culture system. In this technique, early mouse embryos are grown in the laboratory and exposed to various levels of ethanol and antioxidants. Embryos are then monitored for evidence of cell death and abnormal development. "Using this method, we also showed that SOD can diminish ethanol-induced cell death and subsequent malformations," Chen said. As to the new study, Sulik said, the implications apply directly to people with alcoholism. "The nutritional status of alcoholics isn't the best. People who are alcoholic by definition can't control their drinking and often cannot quit drinking during pregnancy. "And so the practical point of this paper is that perhaps we can diminish some of the problems that might exist if the nutritional status of alcoholic mothers improves. It would be great if these women would supplement their diets with a daily multivitamin."

For Women Unable to Quit Drinking

However, just like alcohol, even too many vitamins (especially vitamin A) can be harmful to a fetus, Sulik said. "The idea of possibly adding antioxidants to alcoholic beverages has been proposed as a way of helping the situation, at least a little, for those women who are unable to quit drinking alcohol. "The amount of alcohol used in the study is high, Sulik added, equivalent to the amount that would raise the blood alcohol level of a person up to 0.4 or 0.5. This is a level that can be achieved by chronic alcoholics, people who have acquired a tolerance for alcohol. "Virtually all children born with full-blown fetal alcohol syndrome, with major malformations caused by alcohol, are born to chronic alcoholics," Sulik said. "Chronic alcoholism is a huge problem in our population."

"There is no 'magic number' as to a safe versus unsafe amounts of alcohol consumed during pregnancy," Sulik said. "It would differ from person to person. It would be different depending on the stage of pregnancy, the sensitivity of the developing fetus. "And the stages we're looking at are really very early, before women would even recognize pregnancy. The bottom line: If there's a chance you could become pregnant, don't drink, or if you're drinking don't get pregnant ***END****

CONCLUSIONS
CHANGE WILL COME

"THIS IS TAKEN FROM ONLINE WORK PUBLISHED BY SOMEONE ELSE. I TAKE NO CREDIT FOR THIS WORK... THIS CHAPTER IS CUT AND PASTED FOR THE GOOD OF MANY. If anyone has any issues with that then I will remove it before I launch Edition 1 proper"... Author Henry Africa

START

Billy and Joe

EACH DAY IS UNPREDICTABLE

There are very few places in the country that specialize in residential care for adults with fetal alcohol brain damage. That's what makes Westbrook farm west of Duluth so unique.

It's a gorgeous setting -- 160 acres of rolling pastures and thick forests near the St. Louis River. The farm is home to eight young men struggling with the lasting effects of prenatal alcohol exposure.

WITHOUT THE FARM, HE'D BE IN PRISON

Two brown and white miniature horses nibble hay in the barn. Billy Nelson, 20, gently scratches their ears. Nelson considers the horses his friends -- and his therapy.

"This one's Drummer and that one's Chance," says Nelson. "You can take them out in the yard and run with them, and they stay by your side. They're really nice horses."

Billy Nelson

Nelson has lived at Westbrook for about two years, but it was a rough road getting here. His mom was a drinker. He and his twin brother were born in St. Paul three and a half months premature. His brother died just a few weeks after birth.

Nelson was placed in a series of foster homes, treatment centers and psychiatric care facilities. He was into drugs and alcohol, and was prone to violence. Nelson figures if he hadn't ended up at this farm, he'd probably be in prison.

"I used to be crazy and all that when I first came here, but then I realized what my plan was to do on this earth before I pass on," says Nelson. "I need to take the punches and say, hey, just get my stuff together so I can move on in life and better myself. Because if you don't better yourself, you're not going nowhere. "Westbrook farm was started five years ago by a Duluth non-profit organization called Residential Services, Inc.

The goal is to teach basic living skills to adults affected by fetal alcohol exposure, and help them live independently.

It's a population that health advocates say is grossly underserved in this country. Studies show 90 percent have mental health problems, and 80 percent have trouble holding onto a job.

EACH DAY IS AN EMOTIONAL ADVENTURE

Billy Nelson and the others at Westbrook lack impulse control and have trouble understanding the consequences of their behaviors.

Travis Dombrovski, manager of Westbrook, says that means daily life on the farm is unpredictable and sometimes explosive.

"They break things, and they yell and they scream and they swear, and they're hyper-sexual," Dombrovski says. "Assaults, sure, phones being thrown, lots of property destruction. It's got to be a helpless feeling. It's got to be scary and it's got to be hard to understand."

Travis Dombrovski

Travis Dombrovski says Westbrook's residents have trouble learning from their mistakes, so instead of punishment, they face what he calls "natural consequences." For example, when someone gets angry and breaks something, they're required to fix or replace it.

Despite evidence that punishment is ineffective on adults affected by fetal alcohol, some 60 percent of them will spend time behind bars. Dombrovski say society needs to take a different approach.

"They don't need to be in jail. Jail is not the right place," says Dombrovski. "Sure, there might be structure, but there's no learning, there's no help, there's no support. And it's a waste of a human life, in my opinion, to leave them in jail. They can come out. They can make it."

There's typically a long waiting list to get into Westbrook. Residents are usually referred there by county social service agencies, which pay the costs through foster care and other program funds.

The residents start out living in the main farmhouse, where life is highly structured. They're assigned daily chores. They learn how to cook and clean and take care of themselves. They tend to the farm animals and work in the garden.

Then, when they're ready, they can graduate to more independent living in an apartment building just across the yard.

Billy Nelson says he's ready to move into one of those apartments. For the first time in his life, he's set some goals for himself. He wants to earn his GED, and would someday like to study climatology. Nelson says Westbrook has given him a confidence he's never had before.

"Trust was a big issue when I first came here," says Nelson. "I didn't trust no one. Not even myself. Didn't believe in myself. But now I do believe in myself. And I know I can do whatever I want to, as long as I put my head to it."

Jodee Kulp

Helping alcohol-exposed children grow into adults can be a nightmare for parents. Jodee lives in a western Twin Cities suburb, where she and her husband raised their adopted daughter, Liz, who's now 21 years old.

Jodee says people with more visible disabilities have clear safety nets, but for young adults with FETAL ALCOHOL SYNDROME getting help can be a struggle.
The Kulp family

"The rule is, fail first. And failing first is very painful," says Kulp. "It's very painful as a parent to watch your child fail. It's very painful to watch your child fail over and over and over again."

Like many people with fetal alcoholbrain damage, Liz has trouble managing her money. She's gone into treatment twice for alcohol abuse. Liz says when she first moved out on her own at age 18, one of her biggest problems was housing. She says people took advantage of her.

"I had basically a party house where friends wouldn't leave," Liz says. "By me just inviting maybe one person, they invite whoever else. But they wouldn't leave and then I didn't know what to do, and eventually got kicked out of a lot of apartments."

In all, Liz was booted from nine apartments in just two years. Her mother says Liz tried to do the right thing, but just wasn't capable.

Jodee Kulp says

"For a long time, I felt like I was swimming in the sharks, running around from place to place trying to save her and help her, and try to teach her and help her learn," says Jodee Kulp. "And then finally you look at the situation and say, you know what, in order for her to get services, I've just got to let her fail. And then you just go on your knees, because that's the only option you've got is to just let it happen."

Kulp's daughter eventually qualified for disability services. Liz gets financial help with her rent. The county provides Liz with a job coach to help her find work. She's managed to keep the same apartment for almost a year.

Liz says she still struggles just to contain her emotions. She says little things will irritate her and she can feel the anger welling up in her body. Sometimes it turns into a meltdown, and Liz says things she doesn't mean.

"I can get out of hand. I've calmed down a little bit, but I tend to break things," says Liz. "And people all turn their head and I get frustrated and I yell at them all, because I don't like it when people stare me down. It frustrates me, because they look at me like I'm crazy or something. It's just that I'm frustrated and I don't know how to maintain, and I'm just like, breaking out of my own skin."

"I look at Fetal Alcohol Syndrome as a wicked fountain of youth. Nobody acts the age that they appear to be. You are forever a child."
Monica Adams, an adult with FASD

Jodee Kulp quit her job years ago to devote her life to helping Liz succeed. She helped Liz write a book about what it's like to live with fetal alcohol damage. Liz is now working on a second book focusing on the challenges of making the transition to adult life. Jodee and Liz work together to raise awareness of the disorder.

"The first thing we need to do is we need to change our frame of reference, which is realizing they have a brain injury," says Jodee Kulp. "Once we understand that we're dealing with a brain injury, we start working with the population in a different way... The idea is to build a national voice for persons with fetal alcohol."

What's most difficult for Liz's dad, Karl Kulp, is to not blame Liz for her bad behavior. Karl says he still has to remind himself that Liz can't help it because her brain is damaged.

Karl says the future is too far ahead to even consider that Liz could someday become a productive adult.

"We're immensely gratified that Liz is alive at 21," Karl says. "There were so many ways, and there have been so many instances along the way, where it could have gone the other way and she may not have survived. And it isn't clear yet whether she's going to make 22.

She just doesn't have the brain function to guide herself in the right way all the time. So she makes a lot more mistakes."

Monica Adams

MAKING IT WORK -- WITH HELP FROM OTHERS

Some adults with fetal alcohol damage are doing their best to lead productive lives. Monica Adams is assistant manager of a women's clothing store in a Twin Cities suburb.

"Is there anything I can get for anyone?" says Adams to several customers. "Just looking? OK. If you have any questions, don't hesitate to ask."

Monica at work

Adams, 37, has gone through two failed marriages. Now she's moved back in with her adoptive parents. Adams says she struggled all her life to fit in and understand the world around her. She sucked her thumb habitually until fifth grade. She had no concept of money or time, and school was always frustrating.

"A lot of things I just flat out didn't understand," says Adams. "I mean, a teacher would be talking and I'm like, what in the world is coming out of her mouth? Everybody else seemed to know. I was always the 'day late' person, always asking the person next to me. I feel like I got more of an education adapting to my surroundings than I ever did learning the ABCs, because I had to. "Adams says she's learned to adapt to her disability with strong support from family, friends and an employer who's willing to put up with her faults.

Her boss, store manager Mary Harrell, says she knew a little about fetal alcohol syndrome before Adams told her she had it. Harrell says she and the other store employees are willing to work around Adam's sometimes inconsistent behavior.

Monica and her boss

"Probably the area that I see it the most is the disorganization part of it. We just all work with it," says Harrell. "If we have to clean up after her or, you know, pick things up or rearrange things, I'm willing to sacrifice that, because she's just an incredibly talented, creative person and is great with customers. I guess in any job you're going to have people that do certain things better than others."

Adams says she has a short fuse and works hard to keep her emotions in check. One of her biggest challenges is managing money, and trouble with short-term memory makes that even tougher.

Sometimes she forgets to pay bills, though she's gotten better. She says she's lost track of how many times she's had her driver's license suspended for forgetting to pay insurance or renew her license tabs.

"I mean seriously, if I were to rack up collective damages from fines -- I'm talking everything from legal system fines to credit card debts to cell phone bills, long distance bills -- I'm talking well over $10,000," says Adams.

A 'WICKED FOUNTAIN OF YOUTH'

Adams has become an advocate for others with fetal alcohol brain damage. She's on an advisory board for the Minnesota Organization on Fetal Alcohol Syndrome, and speaks to other young women who are struggling to become adults.

Adams says she used to wonder what she might have become had her biological mother not drunk alcohol while she was pregnant. Now, she just focuses on keeping her life together, and accepting the times when that's not possible.

"People say, 'Oh, you seem so normal. You don't act like you have it,'" says Adams, "and then the next month, I can do something that seems so hare-brained stupid, you can't believe I'm capable of doing that."

Health advocates say that, emotionally, people with fetal alcohol damage often function at half their age. Adams says that's true for her. She says she's figured out how to function as an adult, but she knows that part of her will always be a vulnerable little girl.

"I look at it as kind of a wicked fountain of youth," she says. "Nobody ever looks the age that they appear to be. Nobody acts the age that they appear to be. You are forever a child."

For now, Monica's answer is living at home with her folks. But that doesn't work for everyone. ***END****

POST MORTEM
THE BEATING OF YOUR HEART

Here follows a conversation between author and our Creator. My question I would like to pose is going to be posed by God on my behalf.

HENRY:

AM I REALLY HAPPY WITH THE LIFE YOU HAVE GIVEN ME GOD? SHOULD I HAVE BEEN MORE THAN I AM TODAY? ARE YOU UNHAPPY IF I DID NOT LIVE UP TO YOUR EXPECTATIONS? DID YOU EVEN HAVE EXPECTATIONS OF ME?

GOD ANSWERS:

Go sleep Henry. I will talk to you in the morning. While you are asleep, I will show you what the answer should be to these questions. When you awake then you will know what to write. Simply continue on this at that time...**Its now 01h15 Wednesday morning on the 5th Match 2014 and I really am tired...**

Wednesday 5th March 2014 at 12h30... Never wrote anything about this topic...

Thursday 6th March 2014 at 21h50. I saw that I have not finished this page and went to have something to eat... It's hard to write this part of the book...

Thursday 6th March at 23h30... I am going to sit down and STARE at a blank page if it means finishing this page. I cannot understand how come it is so difficult for me to finish these 2 pages. What is holding me back from just getting it done? What could be so important about this part of the book God? I ask to myself...

"Well Henry...Let me give you my point of view. Write what I have to say and don't think too much about what you feel... This is what I have to say and for once you will simply be a typist for me... So says GOD, the I Am...

I have watched what is happening throughout society Henry. I am saddened by the suffering I see taking place. You have written about things you see but I see it all. I see what every one of 8 billion people sees. I feel what 8 billion people feel. When they laugh then I am happy and when they are sad then are a bit sad too. I will never show you I am sad. Do you think that because I show you when I am angry, I also have to let you know I can be sad too? Do you think I cannot find something funny and laugh with you? When you make a joke and are happy then I can laugh with you... I smile when you smile sometimes... I experience joy when you experience joy too. But you respond to the moment. I see the future and have experienced your joy and sadness way ahead of time and have laughed a long time ago even though I enjoy your moment in time with you...

I see the years of your life stretch into the future. I am ready to defend you when others want to harm you. I can order an angel to wipe out tens of thousands because you are in danger. Does it ever occur to you that on a daily basis I may save so many people from harm that being God is not an easy job, if I put it that way... You are a small part of me like everyone else on the planet. I have breathed life into each and every womb... I have designed each and every child... If I have designed them to be perfect then should not I be the one who is angry when I watch what I have created, being deformed by anyone?

How would you like me to stop this carnage Henry? Don't you think I am angry because of what people do to themselves and to their unborn children? The children are mine Henry. No child is born accept by the will of the I Am... Women are carriers of my children. They carry seeds in their wombs and I give those seeds life. Men do nothing but have fun for a while and if I think they may be of value to the woman I allow them to have children. Unless I breathe life into that egg there is no life. Miscarriages are my choice and mine alone. I decide based on the future if I think a child should be allowed to be born. Then you would understand that if I allow a child to be born then it means that I am happy with the future of the child. I am happy with the way his or her life will grow. Does it make sense that I could allow a FAS child to be born when I have the power to stop the birth? You will call it a miscarriage. I will call it an act of God. And I do act. When I see the future consequences of a life. I can stop evil people from being born and I sometimes do. Other times I have to allow them to be born because there is something they have to discover for the world to be a better place in the future. But I never let evil reign too long do I?

Where is Hitler today? But the Volkswagen lives on doesn't it? You travel by plane because of the dreaded V1 and V2 rocket project that killed millions. Where is Alexander the great? But the roadways are better today than they were then? Where is Genghis Kahn today? I let tiny little Vietnam conquer him. Where is USA today? I let Vietnam conquer them too... Is anyone too big for God to conquer Henry? No! And that is the way it will always be. The way it has always been. The world learns from disaster. The world has airplanes because of the World Wars. The world has nuclear power because of world wars...

I write genetic codes... I write DNA and what does mankind do? They discover what I create. No one has created anything I did not want them to discover. Satan with all his power has to ask me before he can do anything to what is mine. As long as you are one of mine you are going to be just fine. Don't question so many things Henry. Learn to trust me. Sometimes you just have to do what I tell you to. For now that is enough... ... Carry on and finish this book before Sunday. You are doing something that is important to me. Just be obedient and do it the way I am telling you to... You are not always very obedient. I have some issues with you but you know them as well as I do. You need to make some changes where they matter most. The world will evolve and change all the time. I am in control.

What you are doing here is not about you. I am allowing you to do this because you are obedient to my voice. But you are not always obedient...Like most people. They listen only till it gets uncomfortable then they start to do what is easy. That is why we have FAS. Most people know what is right to do or not to do. But they choose to do what is easiest. But remember they always live with the consequences when they do. I am there to help but you need to call out and ask me to help. That is a rule of the battle between good and evil. You have a hotline...USE IT or be a toy with strings that Satan will pull as he pleases. That's the end of our talk for now Henry ..."

INSIDE BACK COVER
LIST OF BOOKS BY AFRICA PUBLISHING Co

- ✓ TEACH ME TO SERVE   By Henry Africa & Vincent Cook
- ✓ CHARACTER OF A WINNER   By Henry Africa
- ✓ SAGA OF CITY PARK   By Henry Africa
- ✓ THE PAM PRETORIUS STORY   BY Henry Africa

- ✓ MEG & SPIKY 1   STAYING HAPPILY MARRIED IS HARD…
- o MEG & SPIKY 2   THE JELLYFISH STORY
- o MEG & SPIKY 3   TEACH ME TO RULE

- o MEG & SPIKY 4   SUCCESS IS ABOUT TIME MANAGEMENT…
- o MEG & SPIKY 5   WOMEN CAN DRIVE 2 YA KNOW
- o MEG & SPIKY 6   RAISING TALENTED, FOCUSSED & POSITIVE KIDS
- o MEG & SPIKY 7   SMART HABITS OF THE MONEY MAKERS

- o MEG & SPIKY 8   THE SUPERCOMPUTER & ITS DRIVER
- o MEG & SPIKY 9   THE LANGUAGE OF A DEVELOPED SPECIES
- o MEG & SPIKY 10   CREATION TO THE RIDE INA BOX

- o MEG & SPIKY 11   PROACTIVE IS DA WORD
- o MEG & SPIKY 12   WHAT DO YOU WANNA BE
- o MEG & SPIKY 13   SO MENI BURGERS, SO LITTLE TIME
- o MEG & SPIKY 14   GETTING 100% IN TESTS & EXAMS

- o MEG & SPIKY 15   OLD FASHIONED LOVE STORY 6 NOVEL SERIES

- ✓ MEG & SPIKY 16   MY CROSS TO BEAR - FETAL ALCOHOL SYNDROME

OUR BOOKS CAN BE FOUND ON AMAZON.COM, KINDLE AND KALAHARI.NET
BOOKS WITH A CIRCLE BEFORE THEM ARE CURRENTLY IN PROCESS

BY HENRY AFRICA

*** YOU HAVE **1** LIFE TO LIVE ***

DON'T MESS UP ANYONE ELSES LIFE BECAUSE YOU DIDN'T GIVE A DAMN or didn't try hard enough…

You can choose to drink or NOT to drink. BUT even if you REFUSE to give it up completely, respect the life growing inside of you and let the drinking go for 9 months. If the child is born deformed and you drank during your pregnancy, you will be eaten alive by your conscience.

You WILL live with REGRET and recrimination for the rest of your life. Your conscience will not let you forget. It will torment you till the day you die. I am speaking from 1st hand experience. The power of your conscience can drive you to think of committing suicide. It is not worth doing DRUGS or ALCOHOL as a pregnant mother.

Besides it is the unborn child's right to be born healthy and free of deformities, if at all humanly possible. It is your right to be able to help that child go through the term of pregnancy with every possible avenue of help to give it a fair chance as it starts a new life. You are the first person in the child's defense system. You are the main protector. You have been given that responsibility by God himself.

A child is born free of sin. A child is guilty of nothing… A child is dependent on you… A child is a gift from God… A child is a treasure in your possession…You were once that child…

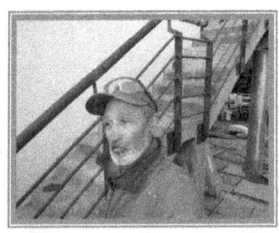

BY HENRY AFRICA

www.ingramcontent.com/pod-product-compliance
Lightning Source LLC
Chambersburg PA
CBHW070259290526
45791CB00003B/1006